DICTIONARY OF
IRIDOLOGY

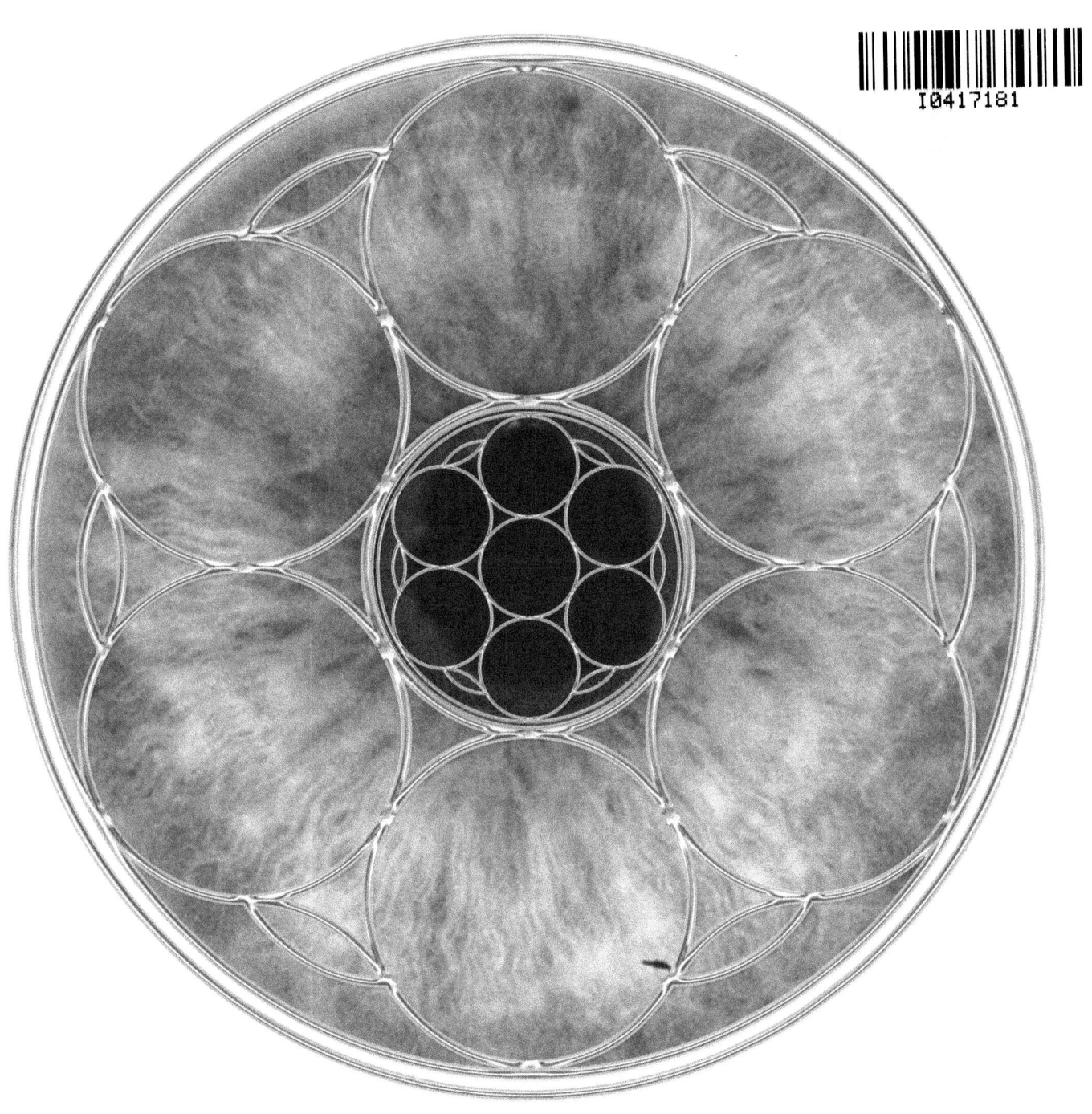

FARIDA SHARAN · GHATFAN SAFI

Wisdome Press
School of Natural Medicine International
www.purehealth.com

Email: faridasharan@purehealth.com
Web: www.purehealth.com
Facebook: www.facebook.com/faridasharan
            www.facebook.com/schoolofnaturalmedicine
Twitter: @healinghumans

Illustrations by Ghatfan Safi ND MIr MH NP MBRI

10 9 8 7 6 5 4 3 2 1

Sharan, Farida & Safi, Ghatfan
      DICTIONARY OF IRIDOLOGY
      ISBN:1511978422

Library of Congress Catalogue
1. Iridology 2. Naturopathy 3. Natural Medicine
4. Healing 5. Health 6. Flower of Life

Printed and bound in the United States of America

Farida Sharan

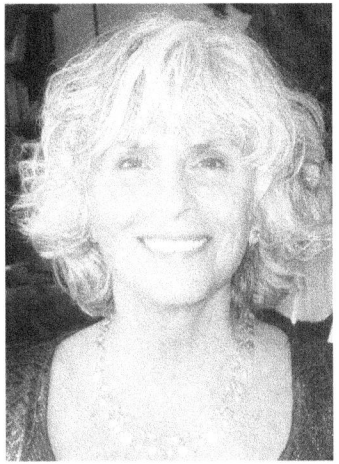

Farida Sharan ND says "My naturopathy teachings of purification, regeneration & transformation evolved after healing breast cancer with natural self-healing. I mentor students to become a living example of the laws of living in life and work — wisdom embodiment — and to share truth as a teacher and guide for those seeking health, healing and wellness.

My first experience with Iridology was when I was told my eyes had turned blue!!! I later learned that the cleansing that had healed breast cancer had released yellow and brown pigments from my iris, and my vision had improved so much, I no longer needed to wear glasses!"

Farida Sharan, ND, is the Founder and Director of the PureHealth School of Natural Medicine, in Boulder, Colorado, an author, educator, natural physician, mystic dancer, yoga teacher, international lecturer and seminar leader.

Her training includes: Esalen massage, Gestalt Therapy, European Massage & Beauty treatments, Reflexology, Shiatsu, Yoga Teacher Training with Yogi Bhajan, Polarity Therapy, Iridology, Naturopathy and Herbal Medicine. Farida received the Master Herbalist Diploma (MH) from Dr. Raymond Christopher and the School of Natural Healing, and Iridology training with Dr. Bernard Jensen. Other trainings include: lymphatic massage, tai chi, chi gong, essential oils, aromatherapy, Flower Remedies with Nora Weeks of the Bach Flower Institute in England, Ashtanga yoga, Living Food Teacher Training & Core Synchronicity cranial bodywork from the New Mexico School of Natural Therapeutics.

Born in Vancouver, Canada where she trained as a gymnast, dancer and yogini, Farida moved to California, USA where she managed art galleries, and health and beauty spas, and trained massage and beauty therapists. After healing breast cancer with Natural Medicine in the early seventies in the Sierra Mountains, at an Essene healing center in southern California, she made Natural Medicine her life work.

From 1977 to 1988 she lived in Cambridge, England, where as a leader in Complementary and Alternative Natural Medicine, she founded the British School of Iridology, the British Register of Iridologists, the premier register honored by the Institute of Complementary & Alternative Medicine in London, and the School of Natural Medicine. During this time she hosted symposiums in Cambridge to bring renowned teachers such as Dr. Bernard Jensen, Dr. Raymond Christopher, Dorothy Hall, Willy Hauser, Harri Wolf and Denny Johnson to present research and create a synthesis of Iridology teachings.

Together with John Morley, she founded Iridology Research and wrote the Iridology Manifesto. She also traveled to Germany to meet with renowned iridologists, Joseph Deck and Willy Hauser, and visit Nature Cure Clinics. In 1986, HarperCollins published her definitive textbook 'Iridology — a Complete Guide to analyzing the colors, textures and markings of the irises of the eye and related forms of treatment'.

Farida was appointed a Director of the *Journal of Alternative and Complementary Medicine* to represent Iridology, awarded a doctorate (MD) from *Medicina Alternativa* in Copenhagen, Denmark, and appointed a Fellow of the Guild of Naturopathic Iridologists. For twelve years in the UK, she worked with patients and students, discovering physical, psychological and spiritual aspects of Iridology and Natural Medicine she shares in her books, teachings and practice.

Travels to India three times a year to visit and teach at the Institute of Naturopathic & Yogic Sciences, yoga ashrams, Ayurvedic clinics and spiritual colonies, enhanced her understanding of the principles of Natural Medicine and Nature Cure. A Natural Physician, Naturopath, Master Herbalist and Iridologist, Farida was in private practice for twenty-five years, several of which were in a gynecological medical clinic in London, England, where client progress was confirmed by medical tests taken before and after treatment. Her associate, Dr. Shirley Bond MD, commented, "I never knew such tissue changes were possible." Farida also received referrals from the Gerson Cancer Clinic and the Bristol Cancer Clinic in England.

A new model of Iridology constitutional types, Transformational Iridology (TI), evolved from years of study, research, practice and teaching. Farida Sharan presented TI to the Guild of Naturopathic Iridologists in Regent's College in London, England in May 2000, the International Iridology Symposium in Sydney, Australia in March 2001, the International Iridology Expo in San Marcos California in June 2002, and the American College of Iridology Conference in Cincinnati, Ohio in October 2002.

Currently residing in Boulder, Colorado, Farida Sharan devotes her life to teaching selected students who choose to receive the wisdom and experience she has to share, in an approved Colorado Department of Higher Education Private Occupational training at Purehealth School of Natural Medicine International.

Ghatfan Safi

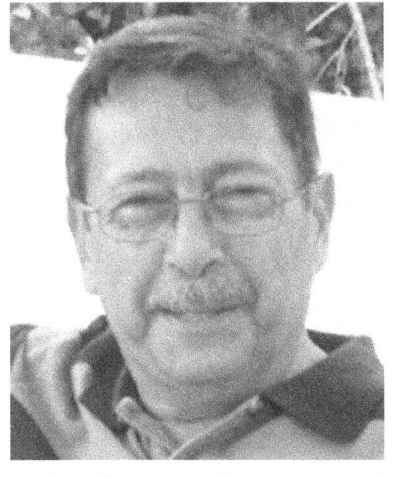

Ghatfan Safi ND MIr MH NP MBRI is the kind of student every teacher dreams about. When he enrolled in the School of Natural Medicine in the UK in the 1980's, his love for Iridology and Natural Medicine was so deep, sincere and enthusiastic, his study exercises of the Iridology & Natural Medicine Online Course materials he was enrolled in created two unique works, *The Iridology Coloring Book* and *The Dictionary of Iridology*.

Ghatfan was born in Lebanon in 1946. He graduated as an architect from the Faculty of Fine Arts in Cairo, Egypt. Shy and introverted, Ghatfan used positive thinking, artistic pursuits, studies and sports to rise above political problems in the Middle East and separation from his family when he worked on building projects in Saudi Arabia.

When Ghatfan graduated from the School of Natural Medicine in Cambridge in 1989, he had healed himself from chronic illness and attained body, mind, spirit transformation, as well remarkable changes in his Iris color. Every student proves the teachings in their own life.

Ghatfan believes in pure Nature Cure and a return to the simple way of life as a cure for disease. His years of practice and teaching in Lebanon prove the success of the teachings as he assisted clients to health, wellness and healing.

When the course was updated a few years ago, Ghatfan wrote: "You may not believe it, Farida, but I want to re-study your revised course of Iridology. I want to deserve the title of Iridologist. Iridology is not an easy science or art. It is a very deep organic art and science."

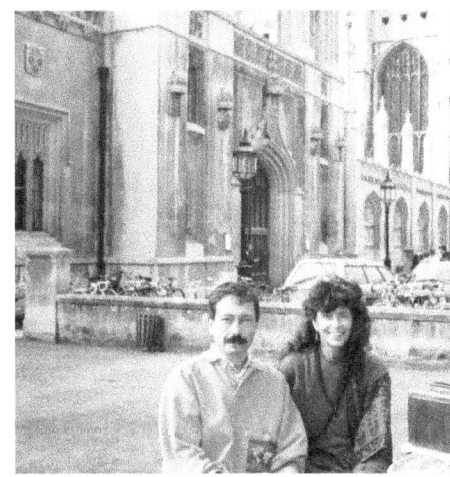

Now retired, Ghatfan devotes himself to his new project, Plantation in Lebanon, in the country near Beirut, where he grows beautiful flowers, and organic fruits and vegetables. Ghafan reports, "The plantation teaches me lot of things about organic gardening which actually needs deep knowledge about how to merge natural and scientific approaches. This merging is deemed inevitable and of value in the coming years."

Thank you, Ghatfan, for your loving appreciation, enthusiasm, creativity, devotion and contribution to the world of Iridology.

Ghatfan Safi and Farida Sharan are shown in the above photograph in front of Kings College, Cambridge during the time Ghatfan graduated as a Naturopath and Master Iridologist in 1989.

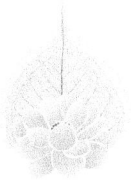

Purehealth School of Natural Medicine

Farida Sharan's teachings of Natural Medicine,
evolutionary self-healing,
and personal transformation
are offered in the
School of Natural Medicine International USA
School of Natural Medicine UK

Iridology and Natural Medicine Online Course (14 lessons)
also includes The Iridology Coloring Book, The Dictionary of Iridology,
Iridology — A Complete Guide (2006 original edition and 2014 revised edition)
as well as Iridology Introduction and Iridology Constitution Seminar Lectures.

Approved Department of Education trainings are offered in:
Naturopathy, Herbal Medicine, Iridology, Reflexology,
Essential Oils, Flower Essences, Healing Diets.

Farida teaches internationally and guides retreats.

Enjoy exploring the websites and blog and email
if you are interested in professional trainings.

Write clearly in the subject line
to make sure we receive your inquiry.

www.purehealth.com
www.herenowhealing.com
www.facebook.com/FaridaSharan
www.facebook.com/SchoolofNaturalMedicine
@healinghumans

faridasharan@purehealth.com

O ABDOMEN (SEE CHART PAGE A13)
O ABDOMINAL WALL (SEE CHART PAGE A13)
O ACIDITY HIGH

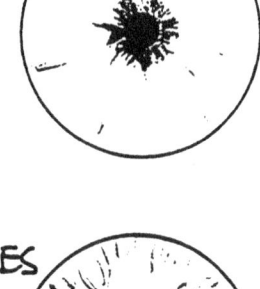

IRIS SIGNS: WHITENESS.

INDICATIONS: OVER ACTIVITY
               CATARRH ACCUMULATION
               INFLAMMATIONS
               ARTHRITIS, BURSITIS, GOUT.
               PAINS, SPASM, KIDNEY STONES
               ACUTE STAGES
               STIFFNESS, BACK ACHE.
               MUCUS FORMATION EXCESS

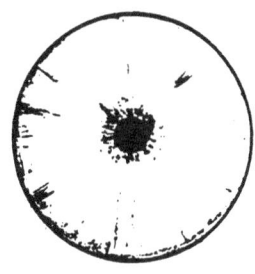

CAUSES: • POOR ELIMINATION
            • HIGH REFINED SUGERS
            • HIGH ANIMAL PROTEINS
            • HIGH DAIRY PRODUCTS
            • SEDATIVE OCCUPATION
            • ACID ALKALINE IMBALANCE
            • POTASSIUM/MAGNESIUM
              IRON, SODIUM, SILICON
              AND IODINE DEFICIENCY.
            • RAW FRESH VEGETABLES
              DEFICIENCY.

WHOLISTIC RELATION SHIPS:

        URINARY & DIGESTIVE SYSTEMS.
        URINARY & CIRCULATORY SYSTEMS.
        DIGESTIVE & RESPIRATORY SYSTEMS.
        DIGESTIVE & CIRCULATORY SYSTEMS.
        MUSCULAR & DIGESTIVE SYSTEMS.
        CIRCULATORY & LYMPHIC SYSTEMS.

TREATMENT :
        BOWELS, KIDNEYS CLEANSING.
        STIMULATE ALL ELIMINATIVE CHANNELS.
        EXERCISE/ SKIN BRUSHING.
        FRESH RAW VEGETABLES FAST
        VEGETABLE BROTH.
        HONEY APPLE CIDER VINAGER.
        ALMONDS, DRIED FIGS, RAISINS, TOMATO JUICE
        VEGAN DIET (STRICTLY).
        MUCUS CLEANSING DIETS
        SUN BATHING, SAUNAS.
        ALKALINE FORMULA (FD)

O ACID STOMACH

IRIS SIGNS : EXTREME WHITENESS
IN STOMACH AREA
WHITE RING AROUND
THE PUPIL
(SEE STOMACH)

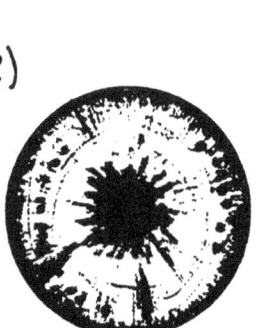

INDICATIONS: OVER ACIDITY
EXCESS HCL SECRETION
HYPERCHLORHYDRIA
EXCESS ACTIVITY OF STOMACH

CAUSES : FAULTY DIET
EXCESS SUGERS
MIXING PROTEINS & STARCHES IN ONE MEAL
ORGANIC SODIUM / CALCUIM DEFICIENCY

WHOLISTIC RELATION SHIPS:
DIGESTIVE & CIRCULATORY SYSTEMS.
DIGESTIVE & URINARY SYSTEMS.
DIGESTIVE & MUSCULAR SYSTEMS.
RESPIRATORY & CIRCULATORY SYSTEMS.

TREATMENT : HIGH ALKALINE DIET.
PROTEINS WITH FRESH RAW VEGETABLES.
GOOD FOOD COMBINATION
HELP GENERAL ELIMINATION.

O ACNE

IRIS SIGNS: WHITENESS.
DARK LIVER AREA (SEE LIVER)
DARK KIDNEY (SEE KIDNEY)
SCURF RIM
LYMPHATIC ROSARY
DARK BOWEL AREA
NERVE RINGS.

INDICATIONS: CONSTIPATION
POOR SKIN FUNCTION
POOR ELIMINATION
TOXIC BLOOD
LYMPHIC CONGESTION
TOXIC BOWELS
OVER LOADED KIDNEY
UNDER FUNCTION LIVER.

CAUSES : HIGH ACIDIC DIET, REFINED SUGERS & DAIRY.
POOR ELIMINATION, RAPID GROWTH.
LIVER CONGESTION, WEAK KIDNEYS,
SLUGGISH SKIN.

ACNE

WHOLISTIC RELATION SHIPS:

               DIGESTIVE & URINARY SYSTEMS
               URINARY & CIRCULATORY SYSTEMS
               CIRCULATORY & RESPIRATORY SYSTEMS
               RESPIRATORY & DIGESTIVE SYSTEMS
               DIGESTIVE & LYMPHIC SYSTEMS

TREATMENT : BOWELS CLEANSING
               BLOOD PURIFICATION
               STIMULATE ALL ELIMINATIVE CHANNELS
               SKIN BRUSHING
               HIGH ALKALINIC DIET
               HERBAL FORMULAE.
               A VITAMIN & ZINC SUPPLEMENTS.

O ACUTE CONDITIONS
(SEE ALSO STAGES OF DISEASE)

IRIS SIGNS:
    RAISED WHITE FIBRES
      IN ORGANS AREAS.

INDICATIONS:
  . HEAVY CATARRHAL
    SETTLEMENT IN
    THE ORGAN AREA
  . ACUTE STAGE OF
    DISEASE.
  . POOR DRAINAGE
  : PAIN
  : INFLAMMATION
  . EARLY STAGE OF
    TOXIC SETTLEMENT.

IRIS A : ACUTE STAGE IN
    ORGAN AREA BLUE IRIS

IRIS B : ACUTE STAGE IN ORGAN
    AREA BROWN IRIS.

IRIS C : ACUTE STAGE OF
    LYMPHIC CONGESTION.

IRIS D : ACUTE STAGE OF BLOOD TOXICITY. ARTHRITIS, RHEUMATISM.

CAUSES: SEE ACIDITY

WHOLISTIC RELATIONSHIP: SEE ACIDITY

TREATMENT: SEE ACIDITY

O ADRENAL GLAND (SEE CHART PAGE A13)

O ALCOHOLISM

IRIS SIGNS: LOSS OF EYE BRIGHTNESS
NERVE RINGS, DILATED PUPIL.
BRAIN ANEMIA
SODIUM RING, DILATED ANW
DARK LIVER AREA
EXTENDED SCURF RIM
FROM LUNG AREA TO SCLERA.
YELLOW-RED-BROWN
TOXIC SETTLEMENTS.
DARK BOWELS AREA
DARK PANCRIAS, DARK THYROID.

INDICATIONS: STRESS
ORGANS EXHAUSTION
POOR ELIMINATION, POOR ASSIMILATION.
ARTERIOSCLEROSIS
OXYGEN STARVATION
B3 VITAMIN DEFICIENCY
B FAMILY & C VITAMINS DEFICENCY
PANCRIATIC EXHAUSTION.

WHOLISTIC RELATION SHIPS:
DIGESTIVE & URINARY SYSTEMS
NERVOUS & CIRCULATORY SYSTEMS
ENDOCRINE & NERVOUS SYSTEMS.

TREATMENT: BOWELS CLEANSING
LIVER FLUSHING
GALL BLADDER CLEANSING
BLOOD PURIFICATION
CASTOR OIL PACKS
RFLEXOLOGY
AVOID STRESS
RELAXTION PROGRAMS & GENTLE EXERCISE.
SEDATIVE HERBAL FORMULAS.
FRUITS JUICE FAST
VEGETABLES BROTH.

O ALIMENTARY CANAL
GASTROINTESTINAL TRACT
- STOMACH.
- SMALL INTESTINES.
- LARGE INTESTINE.
- ESOPHAGUS.
(SEE ALSO DIGESTIVE SYSTEM)

CHART

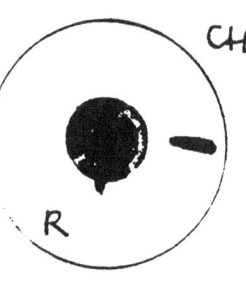
R

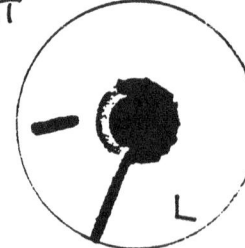
L

O ANEMIA OF BRAIN

IRIS SIGNS: LOSS OF IRIS FIBRES
AT TOP OF THE IRIS.

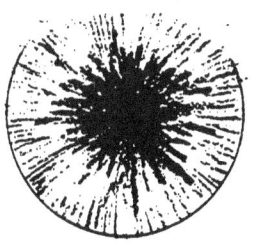

INDICATIONS: POOR CIRCULATION
OXYGEN STARVATION
AGEING
HYPOFUNCTION OF SOME
ORGANS.
POOR IRON ABSORBTION
HAIR GREYING & BALDNESS

CAUSES: OVER EATING
HEAVY MEALS
LACK OF EXERCISE
SEDATIVE LIFE STYLE
POOR BREATHING
REFINED SUGERS
B FAMILY & C VITAMINS DEFICIENCY
E VITAMIN DEFICIENCY
(ABSORBABLE) IRON DEFICIENCY

WHOLISTIC RELATION SHIPS:
CIRCULATORY & RESPIRATORY SYSTEMS
CIRCULATORY & DIGESTIVE SYSTEMS
CIRCULATORY & NERVOUS SYSTEMS

TREATMENT:
TIP-UP SLANT BOARD EXERCISE
WALKING BAREFEET ON SAND OR GRASS
EXERCISE
BLOOD PURIFICATION
STIMULATE CIRCULATION
FRESH RAW FRUITS & VEGETABLES.
E VITAMIN (NATURAL ORGANIC SOURCES)
BREATHING EXERCISE.
ORGANIC IRON RICH FOOD (LEAFY VEGETABLES)

O ANEMIA OF THE EXTREMETIES

IRIS SIGNS: GREYISH-WHITE CAP
IN HEAD AND LEG AREAS

INDICATIONS: LACK OF CIRCULATION.
PLAQUING OF THE
ARTERIAL WALLS.
SODIUM RING DEVELOPMENT.
COLDNESS OF EXTREMETIES.
TENDER SKIN.

CAUSES : POOR BLOOD NOURISHMENT, POOR CIRCULATION.
SEDATIVE LIFE STYLE
LACK OF EXERCISE
COMMERCIAL SODIUM OVER CONSUMPTION.
CHEMICAL IMBALANCES
POOR SKIN ELIMINATION
SUPPRESSED SKIN PERSPIRATION
TOXIC BOWELS

ANEMIA OF THE EXTREMETIES

CAUSES: POOR BREATHING
THYROID HYPOFUNCTION
SMOCKING, AIR POLLUTION
DRUGS THERAPIES

WHOLISTIC RELATIONSHIPS:
CIRCULATORY & RESPIRATORY SYSTEMS.
CIRCULATORY & LYMPHIC SYSTEMS.
CIRCULATORY & ENDOCRINE SYSTEMS
CIRCULATORY & DIGESTIVE SYSTEMS
CIRCULATORY & MUSCULAR SYSTEMS.

TREATMENT:
ANAEMIA FORMULA (ID)
STIMULATE CIRCULATION
HOT & COLD WATER BATHES
BARE FEET WALKING ON SAND AND OR GRASS
BLOOD PURIFICATION
CHEMICAL BALANCES
FRESH RAW FRUITS & VEGETABLES
BOWELS CLEANSING
ORGANIC IRON SUPPLEMENTS
BREWERS YEAST
B VITAMINS, E VITAMIN.
C VITAMIN & BIOFLAVINOIDS.
VEGETABLES (LEAFY) BROTH
WHEAT GERM OIL, LIVER FISH OILS
NATURAL MULTI MINIRALS & VITAMINS HERBAL FORMULA (FI

O ANEMIA RING

IRIS SIGNS: WHITE _ BLUE HAZE
OUTSIDE IRIS RIM

INDICATIONS: POOR CIRCULATION
SKIN UNDER FUNCTION
OXYGEN STARVATION
IRON MALABSORBTION

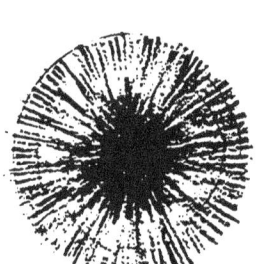

CAUSES: INTESTINAL PARASITIS
POOR ELIMINATION
SKIN UNABLE TO ELIMINATE METABOLIC WASTES
IRON DEFICIENCY
B & C VITAMINS DEFICIENCY
TOXIC BOWELS, TOXIC BLOOD
MAL NUTRITION
BAD LIVING HABITS
BRONCHITIS, ASTHMA, TUBERCULOSIS

WHOLISTIC RELATIONSHIPS:
CIRCULATORY & RESPIRATORY SYSTEMS
CIRCULATORY & LYMPHATIC SYSTEMS
CIRCULATORY & ENDOCRINE SYSTEMS
CIRCULATORY & DIGESTIVE SYSTEMS
CIRCULAORY & MUSCULAR SYSTEMS
CIRCULATORY & URINARY SYSTEMS.

ANEMIA RING
    TREATMENT: SEE ANEMIA OF THE EXTREMETIES

O ANIMATION LIFE (SEE CHART PAGE A13) (SEE NERVOS SYSTEM)

O ANUS (SEE CHART PAGE A13)

O ANXIETY

IRIS SIGNS:
    BROWN SIGNS IN
        INHERIT MENTAL AREA
    NERVE RINGS
    DILATED PUPIL
    DILATED ANW
    DARK BOWELS
    DARK ADRENAL
    SPINAL LESIONS
    RADII SOLERIS
    BROWNISH LUNGS

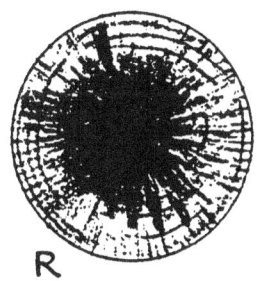 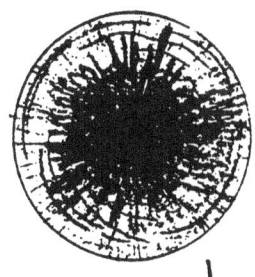

R   L

INDICATIONS:
    HYPERACTIVE OR HYPOACTIVE ADRENALS
    ORGANIC IRRITATION
    METABOLIC IRRITATION
    TOXIC BOWELS, CONSTIPATION, TOXIC BLOOD
    POOR BODY TONE
    POOR BREATHING

CAUSES:
    INHERITED WEAKNESS
    INHERITED LIFESTYLE
    INSOMNIA, SHORT BREATHING
    CHEMICAL IMBALANCES
    ANIMAL PROTEIN EXCESS
    REFINED CARBOHYDRATES EXCESS
    STRESS, SOCIAL ENVIROMENT, FEAR
    ADRENAL IMBALANCE
    CONSTANT DOING, BUISY MIND, CONSTANT ALERT.
    MAGNESIUM & POTASSIUM DEFICIENCY.
    B VITAMIN DEFICIENCY
    DIGESTIVE DISORDERS
    NERVOUS IRRITATION, DEPRESSION
    POOR ELIMINATION.

WHOLISTIC RELATION SHIPS:
        NERVOUS & CIRCULATORY SYSTEMS.
        NERVOUS & DIGESTIVE SYSTEMS.
        NERVOUS & ENDOCRINE SYSTEMS.

TREATMENT:
    BREATHING EXERCISE
    ACID ALKALINE BALANCING
    REFLEXOLOGY
    BOWELS CLEANSING, LIVER FLUSHING, BLOOD PURIFICATION
    BACH FLOWER REMEDIES
    RELAXATION PROGRAMES
    CHELATED MAGNESIUM SUPPLEMENTS
    B VITAMINS SUPPLEMENTS.

O AORTA (SEE CHART PAGE A14)

O APPENDIX (SEE CHART PAGE A13)

O APPENDICITIS

A _ ACUTE APPENDICITIS (BLUE IRIS)
    IRIS SIGNS: RAISED WHITE FIBRES
          IN APPENDIX AREA
          YELLOW-WHITE LYMPHIC
           ROSARY
          WHITE PEYER'S PATCHES
          PSORIC SPOTS
          DARK BOWELS AREA
    INDICATIONS: CONSTIPATION, POOR DIGESTION
          ACUTE LYMPHIC CONGESTION
          APPENDIX INFLAMMATION.

B _ CHRONIC APPENDICITIS (BROWN IRIS)
    IRIS SIGNS: DARK BROWN APPENDIX
    DARK BROWN BOWELS AREA
    BROWN LYMPHIC ROSARY
    PSORIC SPOTS
    NERVE RINGS
    INDICATIONS: CHRONIC CONSTIPATION
          STRESS
          LYMPHIC CONGESTION

C _ APPENDICTOMY (BLUE IRIS)
    IRIS SIGNS: BLACK APPENDIX
          DARKNESS IN CECUM AND
          ASCENDING COLON
          DARK BOWELS AREA
          LYMPHATIC TOPHI

CAUSES:

A _ ACUTE STAGE : CONSTIPATION
          LYMPHIC CONGESTION
          POOR DIGESTION

B _ CHRONIC, DEGENERATIVE STAGE:
          DRUGS SUPPRESSION
          CHRONIC CONSTIPATION
          TOXIC BLOOD, TOXIC BOWELS
          CHRONIC LYMPHIC CONGESTION
          TONSILITIS (SUPPRESSED)
          LAXATIVES

C _ APPENECTOMY:
          CREATS A VERY TOXIC CONDITION IN THE
          ILEOCECAL VALVE, ILEUM & ASCENDING COLON, TOXIC BODY.

WHOLISTIC RELATION SHIPS:
          DIGESTIVE & LYMPHIC SYSTEMS
          DIGESTIVE & NERVOUS SYSTEMS
          DIGESTIVE & MUSCULAR SYSTEMS

TREATMENT: BOWELS CLEANSING/ HERBAL ENEMAS
          CASTOR OIL PACKS
          HIGH FIBRE DIET
          FRESH FRUITS & VEGETABLES
          HIGH ALKALINE DIET

O ARCUS SENILIS (SEE ALSO ANEMIA AT BRAIN)

    IRIS SIGNS: WHITE ARCH ACROSS
               TOP OF IRIS
    INDICATIONS: CEREBRAL ANEMIA
               BRAIN ANEMIA
               LOSS OF VITALITY
    CAUSES   : SEE ANEMIA AT BRAIN
    WHOLISTIC RELATION SHIPS:
          SEE ANEMIA AT BRAIN & EXTREMETIES.
    TREATMENT: SEE ANEMIA AT BRAIN & EXTREMETIES.

O ARM (SEE CHART PAGE A13)
O ARTERIES (SEE CHART PAGE A14)
O ARTERIOSCLEROSIS (SEE SODIUM RING)
O ARTHRITIS (SEE ALSO ACIDITY)
          (SEE ALSO ACUTE CONDITIONS)

    IRIS SIGNS: WHITNESS.
          WHITE ANW.
          (SCURF RIM MAY EXIST)

    INDICATIONS: CATARRHAL SETTLEMENTS
          OVER ACIDITY
          OVER ACID & TOXIC BLOOD
          ACUTE & PAINFULL STAGE

    CAUSES: POOR ELIMINATION
        CONSTIPATION, POOR DIGESTION
        ALKALINE DEFICIENCY
          CALCIUM, POTASSIUM, MAGNESIUM, SODIUM
          IRON, SILICON, IODINE
        REFINED CARBOHYDRATE EXESS
        ANIMAL PROTEIN EXCESS
        DAIRY PRODUCTS EXCESS
        INHERITED.
        POOR SKIN FUNCTION, POOR KIDNEYS & LIVER.
        LACK OF EXCERCISE
        SEDATIVE LIFE STYLE.
        POOR ENDOCRINE GLANDS.

WHOLISTIC RELATION SHIPS:
        CIRCULATORY & ENDOCRINE SYSTEMS
        CIRCULATORY & RESPIRATORY SYSTEMS
        CIRCULATORY & SKELETAL SYSTEMS
        CIRCULATORY & URINARY SYSTEMS
        CIRCULATORY & DIGESTIVE SYSTEMS
TREATMENT:
        BOWELS, KIDNEYS & LIVER CLEANSING
        EXERCISE, STIMULATE ALL ELIMINATIVE CHANNELS
        ALKALINE DIET, POTASSIUM BROTH
        FRESH RAW VEGETABLES
        PANTETHONIC ACID & C VITAMINS SUPPLEMENTS.
        STRICT VEGAN DIET.

○ ASCENDING COLON (SEE CHART PAGE A13)

○ ASSIMILATION RING (SEE CHART PAGE 13)

○ ASTHMA

IRIS SIGNS:
DARK LUNGS AREA, RADII SOLARIS
WEAKNESS LESION
 AT MEDULLA AREA, RADII SOLARIS
DARK ADRENALS.
UNDR ACID STOMACH.
PSORIC SPOTS, LYMPH ROSARY.
NERVE RINGS.
DARK BOWELS AREA.
SCURF RIM

INDICATIONS:
POOR ELIMINATION, CONSTIPATION.
UNDER FUNCTION MEDULLA (INHERITED)
POOR BREATHING
EXHAUSTED LUNGS
ENDOCRINE HYPOFUNCTION
TOXICITY

CAUSES:
SUPPRESSED BRONCHITIS BY ANTIBIOTICS
INTESTINAL PARASITIS (ASCARIS WORMS)
POOR BREATHING HABITS
SPINAL & CERVICAL LESIONS
POOR RESPIRATION & CIRCULATION, ANEMIA.
LYMPHIC CONGESTION
REFINED CARBOHYDRATES EXCESS
SATURATED FATS EXCESS
TOXIC BLOOD, MUCUS ACCUMULATION
POLLUTION
FRUSTRATIONS, STRESS, IRRITATION
CONTAMINATED OCCUPATION
CONSTIPATION

WHOLISTIC RELATIONSHIPS:
RESPIRATORY & CIRCULATORY SYSTEMS
RESPIRATORY & DIGESTIVE SYSTEMS
RESPIRATORY & ENDOCRINE SYSTEMS
RESPIRATORY & URINARY SYSTEMS
RESPIRATORY & LYMPHIC SYSTEMS
RESPIRATORY & NERVOUS SYSTEMS

TREATMENT:
BLOOD PURIFICATION(Dr.C), BLOOD CIRCULATION (FD)
BOWELS CLEANSING
C VITAMINS
GARLIC, PROPOLIS, NATURAL ANTIBIOTICS (FD)
MUCUS CLEANSING DIETS (POTASSIUM BROTH)
ASTHMA HERBAL FORMULA (FD)
CASTOR OIL PACKS
STIMULATE ELIMINATION

O ATROPHY

IRIS SIGNS:
   GREY BROWN STREAKS
   BROWNISH DISCOLORATIONS
   FIBRE LESIONS.

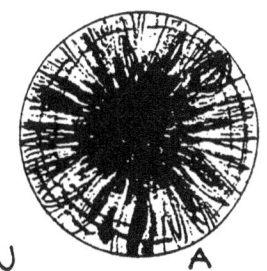 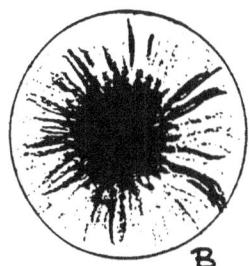

INDICATIONS:
   ABSENT FUNCTION OF THE ORGAN
   INABILITY TO ELIMINATE
   INABILITY TO ABSORB NUTRIENTS
   METABOLIC IRRITATION
   INHERITED WEAKNESS
   UNDER-SIZE OF THE ORGAN

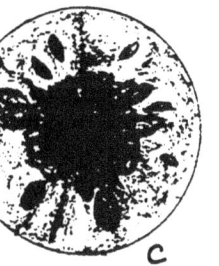 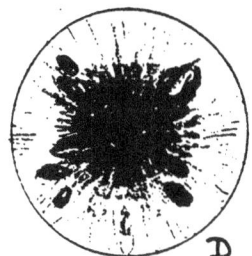

CAUSES:
   CLOGGED CIRCULATION & LYMPH
   LACK OF EXCERCISE
   NERVOUS TENSION
   CHEMICAL IMBALACE
   POOR BODY TONE
   TOXICITY, CONSTIPATION
   SOME ANAEMIC CONDITIONS.

WHOLISTIC RELATION SHIPS,
   ALL SYSTEMS INVOLVED

TREATMENT:
   DEPENDS UPON THE NATURE OF THE ORGAN

ILLUSTRATIONS:
   A — GREY IRIS (RIGHT)
       WEAK CONSTITUTION
       ATROPHY SIGNS AT LEG & RIGHT SHOULDER
   B — BLUE IRIS (LEFT)
       LYMPHATIC TYPE
       ATROPHY SIGNS AT LEFT ARM & SHOULDER
   C — BROWN IRIS (RIGHT) MALE
       WEAKNESS LESIONS
       ATROPHY SIGNS AT SEXUAL ORGANS
        INDICATES: UNDER SIZE PENIS & TESTICLES
                   IMPOTENCE.
   D — BLUE IRIS (RIGHT)
       WEAK CONSTITUTION
       ATROPHY SIGNS AT SPINAL CHORD & NECK AREAS
        INDICATES: POOR POSTURE
                   POOR ALIGNMENT

O AUTONOMIC NERVOUS SYSTEM
(SEE NERVOUS SYSTEM)

O AUTONOMIC NERVE WREATH

* ANW_ AUTONOMIC NERVE WREATH
INDICATES THE:
AUTONOMIC NERVOUS
SYSTEM.

* SNS_ SYMPATHETIC
NERVOUS SYSTEM

* PNS_ PARASYMPATHETIC
NERVOUS SYSTEM

* CNS_ CENTRAL NERVOUS
SYSTEM

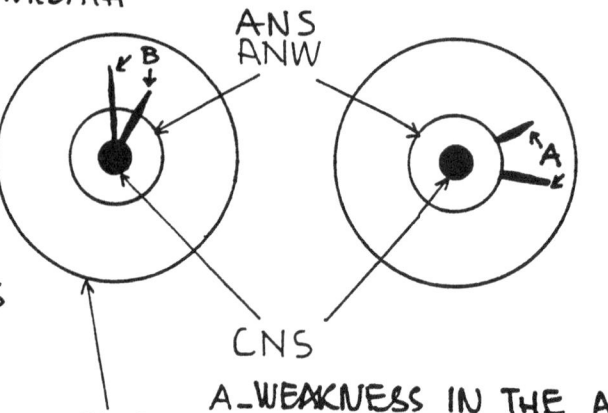

A_ WEAKNESS IN THE ANS
B_ WEAKNESS IN THE CNS

O AUTONOMIC NERVE WREATH ABNORMALITIES
(SEE DIGESTIVE SYSTEM)

A_ CIRCULAR TIGHT ANW
INDICATES: TENSION
AND GOOD CONSTITUTION

B_ STRICTURE
INDICATES: SPASMIC COLON
AND DIGESTIVE DISORDERS

C_ THE UPPER PART BENDED
TOWARDS THE PUPIL
INDICATES: PROLAPSUS
LACUNES INDICATE POCKETS
AND DIVERTICULAE

D_ DILATED ANW
INDICATES VERY POOR
BODY TONE, FEAR
AND EXHAUSTION.

E_ (LEFT IRIS) ANW ENLARGED
AT RIGHT SIDE OF THE IRIS
INDICATES: BALLOONED
DESCENDING COLON AND
CONSTIPATION.

F_ ANW PULLED TOWARDS
PUPIL (RIGHT IRIS)
INDICATES: ABNORMALITY
IN LIVER & GALL BLADDER

G_ BREAKS IN ANW_ CRYPTS OR
RADII SOLARIS BREAK THROUGH ANW
INDICATES: A SERIOUS UNDER FUNCTION
OF THE AUTONOMIC NERVOUS SYSTEM.

H_ RADII SOLERIS OR CRYPTS RADIATING FROM
ANW INTO BODY ORGANS INDICATE:
DISEASE OF ORGANS CONTROLLED BY ANS
LIKE LIVER, KIDNEYS, STOMACH, LUNGS ECT.

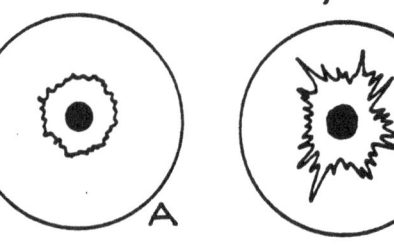
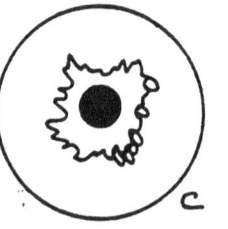
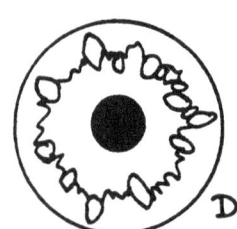
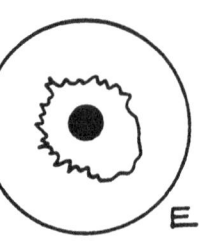
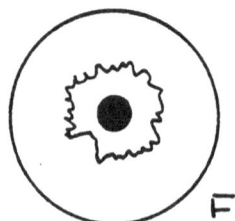
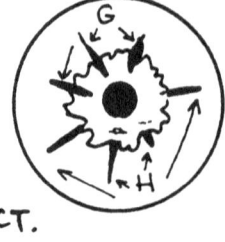

* CHART TO IRIDOLOGY

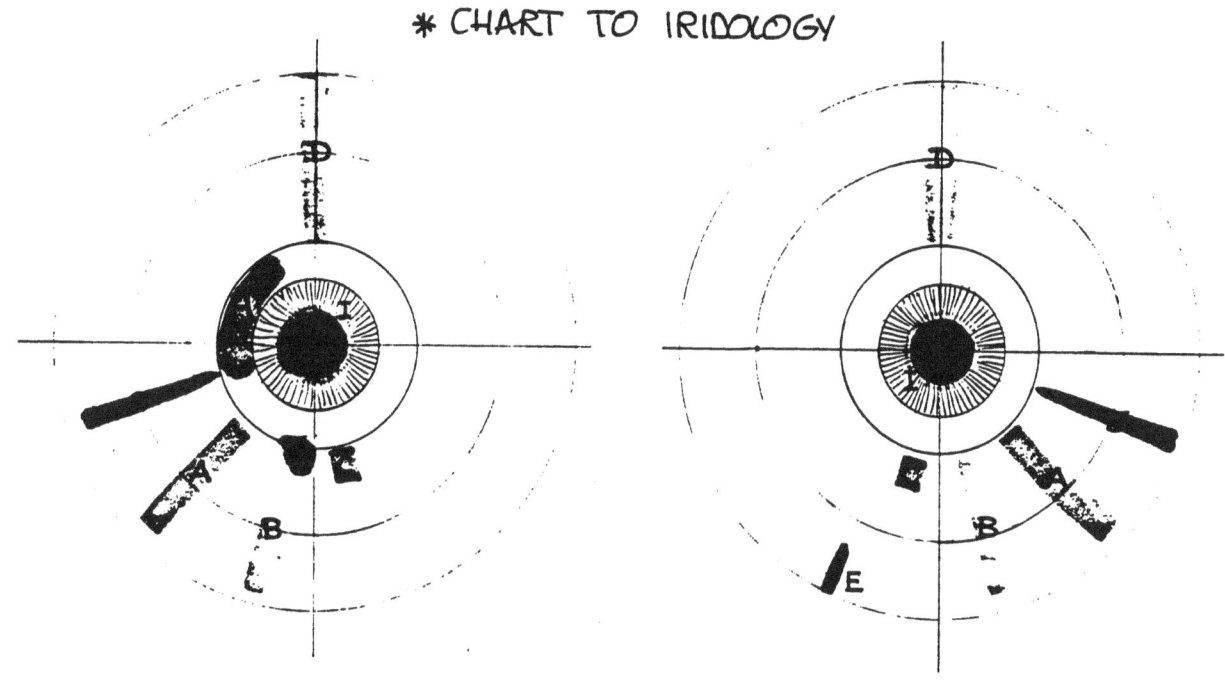

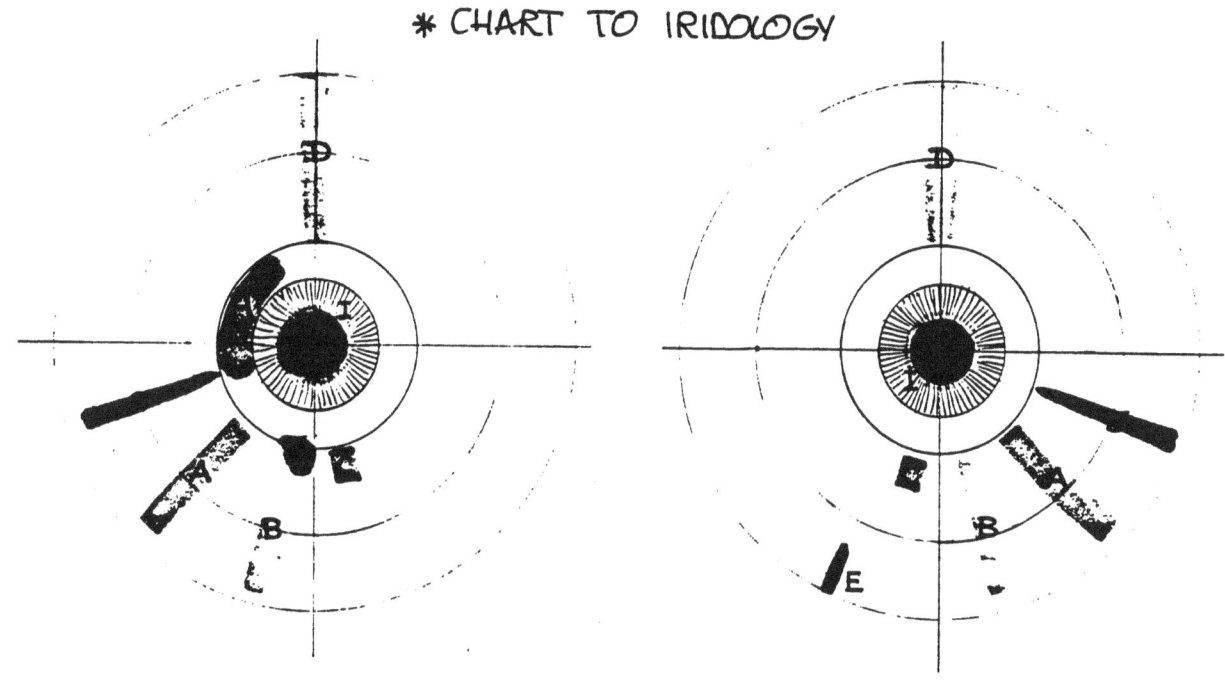 UPPER ABDOMEN
 ABDOMINAL WALL
 ADRENAL GLAND
 ANIMATION LIFE CENTER
 ANUS
 APPENDIX
 ARM

 ASCENDING COLON
 ASSIMILATION RING

* BASED ON CHARTS TO IRIDOLOGY DEVELOPED BY Dr. BERNARD JENSEN AND DOROTHY HALL.

✱ CHART TO IRIDOLOGY

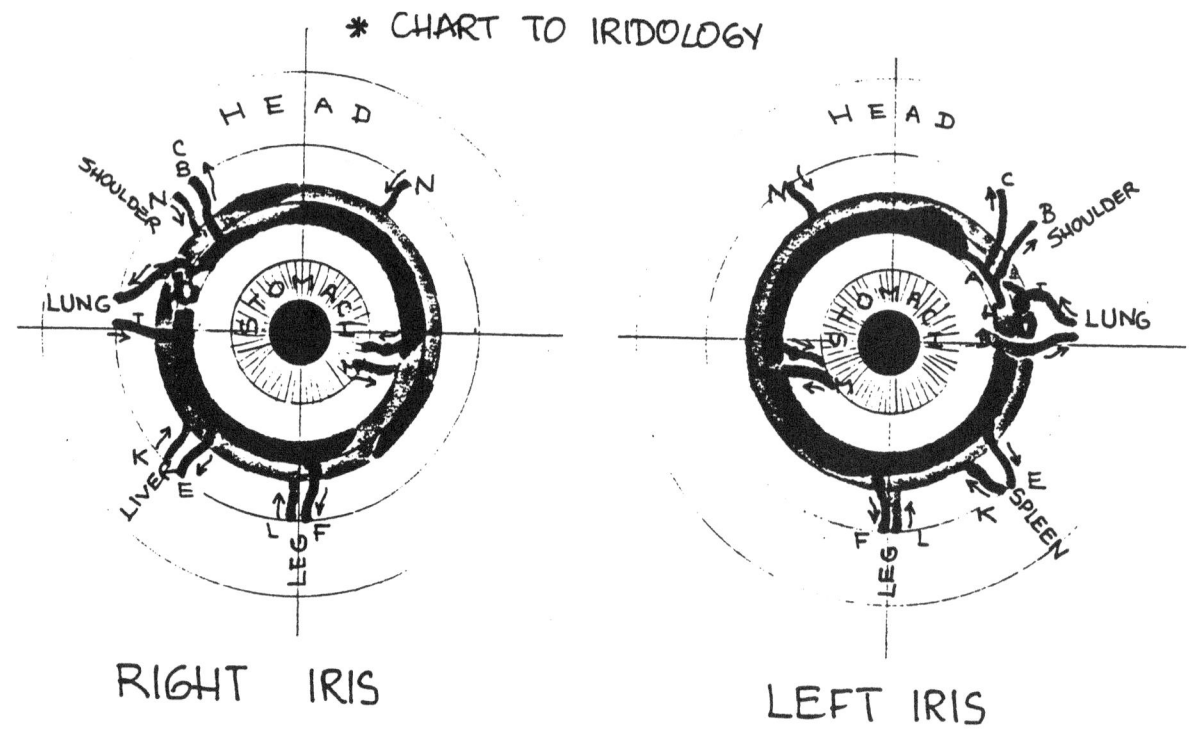

RIGHT IRIS   LEFT IRIS

█ ARTERIAL BLOOD
▪ VENOUS BLOOD

○ A : AORTA
○ ARTERIES:
        G: GASTRIC ARTERY
        D : PULMONARY ARTERY
B : ARTERIAL SUPPLY TO ARM
C : ARTERIAL SUPPLY TO HEAD
E : ARTERIAL SUPPLY TO LIVER (RIGHT IRIS) & SPLEEN (LEFT IRIS)
F : ARTERIAL SUPPLY TO LEGS
I : PULMONARY VEIN
M : GASTRIC VEIN.
N : VENOUS SUPPLY FROM HEAD
K : VENOUS SUPPLY FROM LIVER (R) & SPLEEN (L)
L : VENOUS SUPPLY FROM LEGS.
H : HEART

(SEE ALSO CIRCULATORY SYSTEM PAGE C7)

✱ BASED ON FUNDAMENTAL BASIS OF IRISDIAGNOSIS
   BY THEODOR KRIEGE

O BACK AREA (SEE CHART PAGE B13)

O BACK CONDITIONS (SEE ALSO SKELETAL SYSTEM)

IRIS SIGNS:
WEAKNESS LESIONS
IN BACK AREAS.
DISCOLORATION IN BACK
AREAS, & ENDOCRINE GLANDS
SCURF RIM
TOXIC SETTLEMENTS
NERVE RINGS

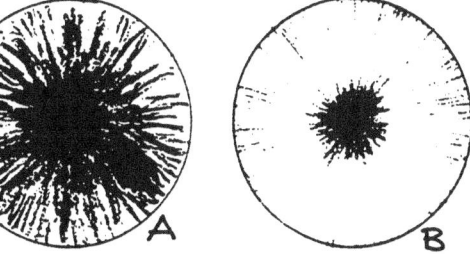

A - GREEN EYE RIGHT IRIS
DARK BACK AREA
POOR BODY CONSTITUTION
TOXIC SETTLEMENTS

INDICATES: POOR POSTURE
POOR ALIGNMENT
CALCIUM DEFICIENCY.

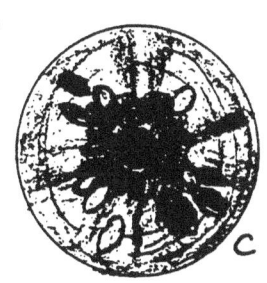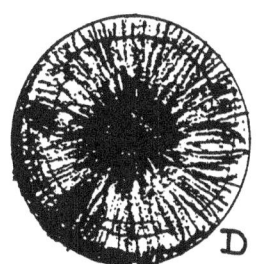

B - BLUE EYE LEFT IRIS
WHITE BACK AREA, TIGHT ANW
WHITENESS, WHITE PITUITARY GLAND
INDICATES: TENSION, STIFFNESS, PAIN & BACK INFLAMMATION

C - BROWN EYE RIGHT IRIS
WEAKNESS LESIONS IN BACK AREAS & NECK.
NERVE RINGS, DARK THYROID AREA.
INDICATES: METABOLIC IRRITATION ENDOCRINE HYPOFUNCTION.
VERY POOR ALIGNMENT, WEAK POSTURE

D - GREY EYE LEFT IRIS
VERY DARK BACK AREA, SCURF RIM, TOXIC THYROID
TOXIC SETTLEMENTS NERVE RINGS.
INDICATES: CHRONIC SPINAL INFLAMMATION
POOR METABOLISM, TOXIC SKELETON
CALCIUM MAGNESIUM DEFICIENCY, ENDOCRINE IMBALANCE.
POOR ELIMINATION.

CAUSES: INHERITED, POOR ENDOCRINE FUNCTIONS.
CALCIUM DEFICIENCY
PHOSPHOROUS, CALCIUM MAGNESIUM IMBALANCE
BAD DIETERY HABITS
BAD SITTING & LIVING HABITS
LACK OF EXCERCISE
STRESS, DEPRESSION.

WHOLISTIC RELATION SHIPS.
SKELETAL & NERVOUS SYSTEMS
SKELETAL & CIRCULATORY SYSTEMS
SKELETAL & ENDOCRINE SYSTEMS
SKELETAL & DIGESTIVE SYSTEMS

BACK CONDITIONS

TREATMENT: CHIROPRACTICE
OSTEOPATHY
ALEXANDER TECHNIQUE
Dr. CHRISTOPHER'S BONE, FLESH, CARTILEGE
   FORMULA.
CALCIUM FORMULA (FD)
THYROID FORMULA
BLOOD PURIFICATION
ENHANCE CIRCULATION
PHOSPHOROUS, CALCIUM & MAGNESIUM BALANCING
STIMULATE ELIMINATIVE CHANNELS
BOWELS CLEANSING.
SUN BATHING
WALKING
EXCERCISE UNDER PROFESSIONAL SUPERVISION.

O BALDNESS

IRIS SIGNS: ARCUS SENILIS. (SEE PAGE A9)
SCURF RIM.
ENDOCRINE DISCOLORATION.
PSORIC SPOTS.
NERVE RINGS.
LIVER, KIDNEYS & SPLEEN
   DISCOLORATIONS.
DARK BOWELS AREA
DARK ASSIMILATION RING
LYMPHIC ROSARY

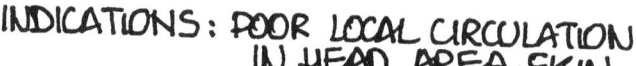

INDICATIONS: POOR LOCAL CIRCULATION
   IN HEAD AREA, SKIN
   & SCALP.
TOXIC BLOOD
TOXIC BOWELS
NERVE IRRITATION
POOR NUTRIENTS ASSIMILATION
THYROID HYPOFUNCTION
LIVER CONGESTION
LYMPHIC CONGESTION
POOR SKIN FUNCTION
STAGNANT URINATION

CAUSES: B VITAMINS DEFICIENCY.
E VITAMIN DEFICIENCY.
REFINED FOODS EXCESS.
ENDOCRINE IMBALANCES, HYPER OR HYPO_ THYROIDISM
LIVER KIDNEYS & SPLEEN UNDERFUNCTION.
LACK OF AIR & SUN EXPOSURE.
OVER EXPOSURE TO SUN & AIR.
TESTOSTERONE EXESS
INHERITED THICKENING OF GALEA APONEUROTICA.
CIRCULATORY & LYMPHATIC POOR CIRCULATION.

BALDNESS

WHOLISTIC RELATIONSHIPS

    CIRCULATORY & MUSCULAR SYSTEMS
    CIRCULATORY & LYMPHIC SYSTEMS
    CIRCULATORY & ENDOCRINE SYSTEMS
    CIRCULATORY & DIGESTIVE SYSTEMS
    CIRCULATORY & URINARY SYSTEMS
    CIRCULATORY & RESPIRATORY SYSTEMS

TREATMENT:

    SLANT BOARD TIP-U-UP EXERCISE
    BOUNCING
    STIMULATE CIRCULATION
    MAGNETIC THERAPY
    THYROID FORMULA (FD)
    ADRENAL FORMULA (FD)
    NATURAL MULTI MINERAL & VITAMINS HERBAL FORMULA (FD)
    WHEAT GERM OIL, FISH LIVER OIL
    BOWELS & BLOOD CLEANSING.
    LIVER FLUSH, GALL BLADDER CLEANSING.

O BALLOONED BOWELS

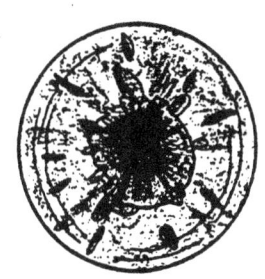

    IRIS SIGNS:
    DILATION OF ANW AT DESCENDING
    COLON & SIGMOID AREAS.

    INDICATIONS:
      BALLOONED DESCENDING COLON
      COLITIS
      CHRONIC CONSTIPATION

    CAUSES:
      SEE CONSTIPATION

    WHOLISTIC RELATIONSHIPS:
      DIGESTIVE & MUSCULAR SYSTEMS
      DIGESTIVE & LYMPHIC SYSTEMS.

    TREATMENT:
      ULTIMATE CLEANSING PROGRAME (Dr. BERNARD JENSEN)
      RECTAL BOLUS (FD)
      HERBAL ENEMAS
      HIGH FIBRE DIET
      EXERCISE

O BLADDER (SEE CHART PAGE B13)
O BLADDER CONDITIONS

IRIS SIGNS:

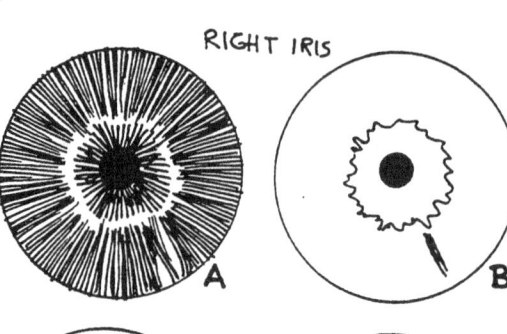

RIGHT IRIS

A _ WHITENESS IN PENIS &
BLADDER AREA.
INDICATES: ACUTE
CYSTITIS / PAIN
AND BURN URINATION.

B _ DARK COLOURS IN
BLADDER AREA
INDICATES: HYPOFUNCTION
AND TOXINS IN BLADDER

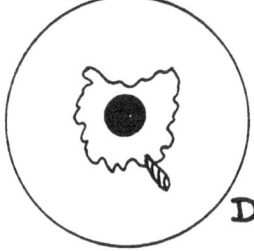

C _ LACUNAE EXTENDED
INTO THE FIFTH ZONE
(SEE ZONES PAGE   )
INDICATE: THE POSSIBILITY
OF CYSTIC PARALYSIS.

D _ PROLAPSUS (SEE ANN
ABNORMALITIES PAGE A12)
INDICATES: BLADDER UNDER SIZE
AND SUPPRESSED FUNCTION

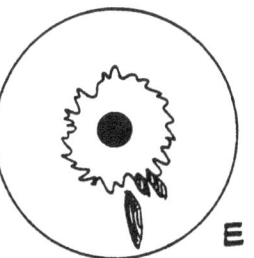

E _ DARK KIDNEY & DARK BLADDER
AREAS
INDICATE: KIDNEY STONES IN BLADDER
AND KIDNEY

NOTE: SCURF RIM / LYMPHATIC ROSERY MAY EXIST.
CAUSES:

(SEE KIDNEY DISEASE)
POOR HYGIENE (FEMALES) DUE TO THEIR SHORT
UTERUS, MAY HELP BACTERIA TO SEEP FROM ANUS INTO
THE VAGINA.
SEXUAL ACTIVITY.
SPINAL LESIONS T6 TO COCCYX.
LIVER CONGESTION.
POOR CIRCULATION.
INADEQUATE FLUIDS IN DIET.
FABRIC UNNATURAL UNDER WEAR & LACK OF PROPER
VENTILATION TO ANUS & VAGINA (FEMALES)
PROLAPSED TRANSVERSE COLON
POOR ELIMINATION, CONSTIPATION

WHOLISTIC RELATIONSHIPS:
URINARY & CIRCULATORY SYSTEMS
URINARY & NERVOUS SYSTEMS
URINARY & SKELETAL SYSTEMS
URINARY & DIGESTIVE SYSTEMS

TREATMENT: (SEE KIDNEY DISEASE TREATMENT)

O BLOOD CIRCULATION
(SEE ALSO CIRCULATORY SYSTEM C7)

CHART

- BLOOD CIRCULATION
SUPPLY STAGE
(SEE CHART PAGE A 14)
THIS IRIS AREA INDICATES:
THE QUALITY OF
ABSORBED BLOOD
FROM SMALL INTESTINES
INTO THE BLOOD
STREAM.

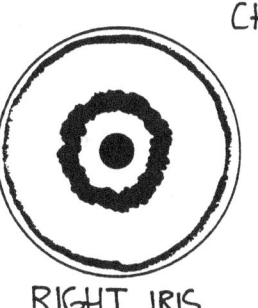 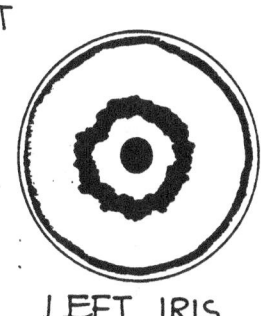

RIGHT IRIS   LEFT IRIS

- BLOOD CIRCULATION
IN MUSCULAR TISSUES AND CAPILLARIES
THIS IRIS AREA INDICATES: THE QUALITY OF CIRCULATION
AT THE EXTREMETIES AND ANEMIA CONDITIONS
(SEE ANEMIA)

O BLOOD CIRCULATION CONDITIONS
SEE ALSO ACIDITY, SODIUM RING, RADII SOLERIS

A — WHITENESS, SCURF RIM
INDICATES: CATARRHAL
ACCUMULATION & MUCUS
EXCESS DUE TO ACIDIC BLOOD
CONDITION.

B — YELLOW & RED CIRCULATION
AREAS INDICATE DRUGS LADENED
BLOOD STREAM.

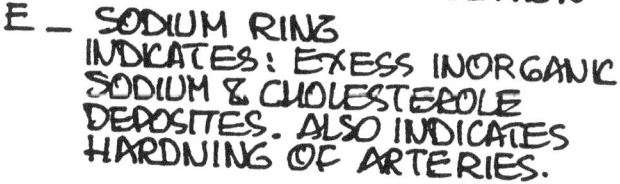

C — RADII SOLERIS BREAKING THE ANW
LEGS, LUNGS, HEAD AND OTHER
ORGANS. INDICATE: TOXIC BLOOD
SEEPING INTO ORGANS & LEG
CAUSING VARICOSE VEINS.

D — ARCUS SENILIS & ANEMIA AT
THE EXTREMETIES.
INDICATES: POOR CIRCULATION

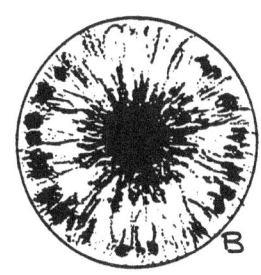
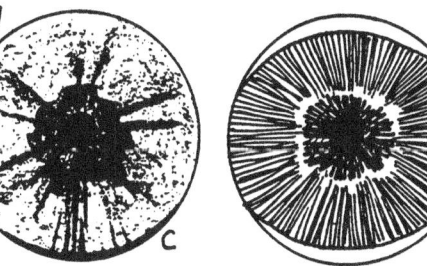

E — SODIUM RING
INDICATES: EXCESS INORGANIC
SODIUM & CHOLESTEROLE
DEPOSITES. ALSO INDICATES
HARDNING OF ARTERIES.

F — DARK ANW & DARK SCURF
RIM.
INDICATE: A SERIOUS CONDITION
OF BLOOD TOXICITY & POOR
BLOOD CIRCULATION. THIS CASE
LEAD EVENTUALLY TO A FATAL CONDITION.

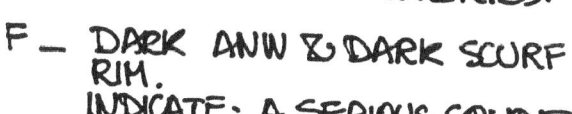
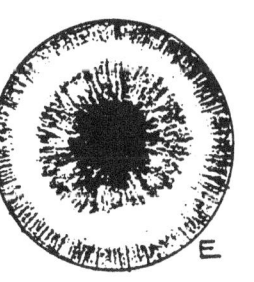
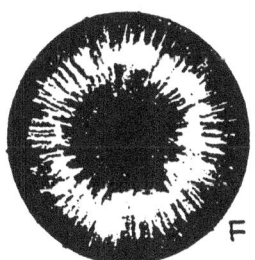

CAUSES: SEE CIRCULATORY SYSTEM
WHOLISTIC RELATIONSHIPS: SEE CIRCULATORY SYSTEM.
TREATMENT: SEE CIRCULATORY SYSTEM.

O BLOOD PRESSURE AREA (SEE CHART PAGE B13)

O BLOOD PRESSURE CONDITIONS (HIGH)

IRIS SIGNS:

A _ RAISED WHITE LINES IN THE EGO
PRESSURE AREA
INDICATES: HIGH BLOOD PRESSURE

B _ SODIUM OR CHOLESTEROLE RING
INDICATES: HIGH CONSUMPTION OF NON
ORGANIC SODIUM, ARTERIOSCLEROSIS.
AND CHOLESTEROLE DEPOSITES ON
ARTERY WALLS WHICH ALL LEAD TO
HIGH BLOOD PRESSURE.

C _ GOOD CONSTITUTION, TIGHT ANW
SMALL PUPIL.
INDICATES: A HEALTHY LOOKING BODY
BUT VERY TIGHT AND TENSIONED
AUTONOMIC NERVOUS SYSTEM, WHICH
LEAD TO HYPERTENSION.

D _ POOR CONSTITUTION, WHITNESS
LYMPHIC ROSARY
INDICATES: POOR BODY TONE
POTASSIUM, MAGNESIUM AND CALCIUM
DEFICIENCY WHICH LEAD TO
HIGH BLOOD PRESSURE

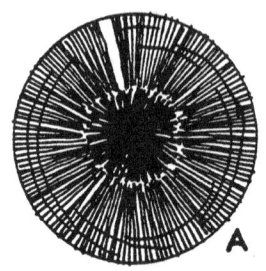
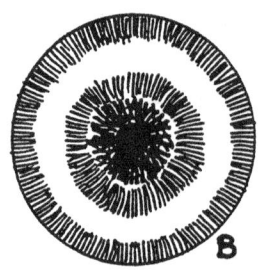
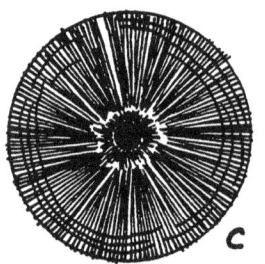
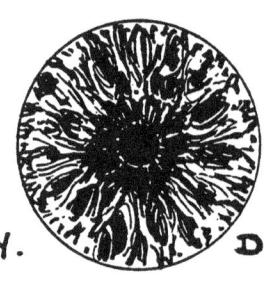

CAUSES:

INCREASED CARDIAC OUT PUT
INCREASED VISCOSITY OF THE BLOOD
INCREASED PERIPHERAL RESISTANCE
OR NARROWING OF THE BLOOD VESSELS
NARROWING OF THE BLOOD VESSELS
CAUSED BY CHOLESTEROLE DEPOSITS
INSIDE THE ARTERIES WALLS.
SODIUM EXCESS
SATURATED FATS EXCESS
PROTEIN EXCESS, DAIRY EXCESS
RFINED CARBOHYDRATES, FIBRE DEFICIENCY.
CANNED FOOD PROCESSED MEATS
PHOSPHOROUS EXCESS
CALCIUM, POTASSIUM & MAGNESIUM DEFICIENCY
E VITAMINE DEFICIENCY OR EXCESS
B & C VITAMINES DEFICIENCY
RAW FRESH VEGETABLES & FRUITS DEFICIENCY
FRIED FOODS, ROASTED NUTS
STRESS.
LACK OF PHYSICAL EXERCISE.
OBESTY, OVER WEIGHT, ODEMA
POOR ELIMINATION, SLOW KIDNEY FUNCTION

BLOOD PRESSURE

WHOLISTIC RELATION SHIPS

CIRCULATORY & NERVOUS SYSTEMS
CIRCULATORY & LYMPHIC SYSTEMS
CIRCULATORY & DIGESTIVE SYSTEMS
CIRCULATORY & RESPIRATORY SYSTEMS
CIRCULATORY & URINARY SYSTEMS

TREATMENT:
VEGAN DIET
ESSENTIAL FATTY ACIDS
POTASSIUM BROTH, LEAFY VEGETABLE BROTH, GARLIC
LECITHIN
WHEAT GERM OIL
WALKING
BLOOD CIRCULATION HERBAL FORMULA (FD)
STIMULATE ELIMINATION

AVOID:
FRIED FOOD
CANNED SALTED FOOD
ROASTED SALTED NUTS
REFINED CARBOHYDRATES
COFFEE, TEA,
STRESS

O BLOOD SUGER (SEE DIABETES)
O BOILS

IRIS SIGNS:
DARK BOWELS AREA
YELLOW_ORANGE ANW
WHITENESS
SCURF RIM
BROWN LIVER AREA, THYROID
NERVE RINGS, PSORIC SPOTS
LYMPH ROSARY

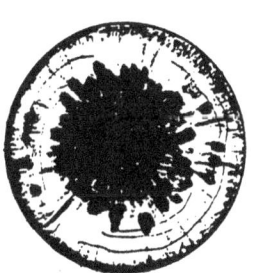

INDICATIONS:
CONSTIPATION
TOXIMIA, TOXIC BLOOD CIRCULATION
SULPHER EXCESS IN BLOOD SUPPLY
POOR SKIN FUNCTION
LIVER CONGESTION
ENDOCRINE IMBALANCES
ACIDITY
LIMPHIC CONGESTION

CAUSES:
REFINED CARBOHYDRATE EXCESS, FIBRE DEFICIENCY.
SATURATED FATS EXCESS, CANNED FOOD EXCESS.
ANIMAL SOURCES PROTEIN EXCESS.
SULPHER DRUGS THERAPY.
POLLUTION, SULPHER POLLUTION.
SLOW ELIMINATIVE CHANNELS.
POOR SKIN FUNCTION

BOILS

CAUSES CONTINUE

RAW FRESH VEGETABLE DEFICIENCY
ALKALINIC FOOD DEFICIENCY
LACK OF PROPER BODY VENTILATION

WHOLISTIC RELATION SHIPS:

CIRCULATORY & DIGESTIVE SYSTEMS
CIRCULATORY & LYMPHIC SYSTEMS
CIRCULATORY & ENDOCRINE SYSTEMS
CIRCULATORY & RESPIRATORY SYSTEMS

TREATMENT:

BOWELS CLEANSING.
BLOOD PURIFICATION.
LIVER FLUSHING & GALL BLADDER CLEANSING.
SKIN BRUSHING.
ACID ALKALINE BALANCING DIET.
VEGAN DIET.

O BONE AREA & BONE DISEASES
(SEE SKELETAL SYSTEM)

O BOWELS AREA CHART

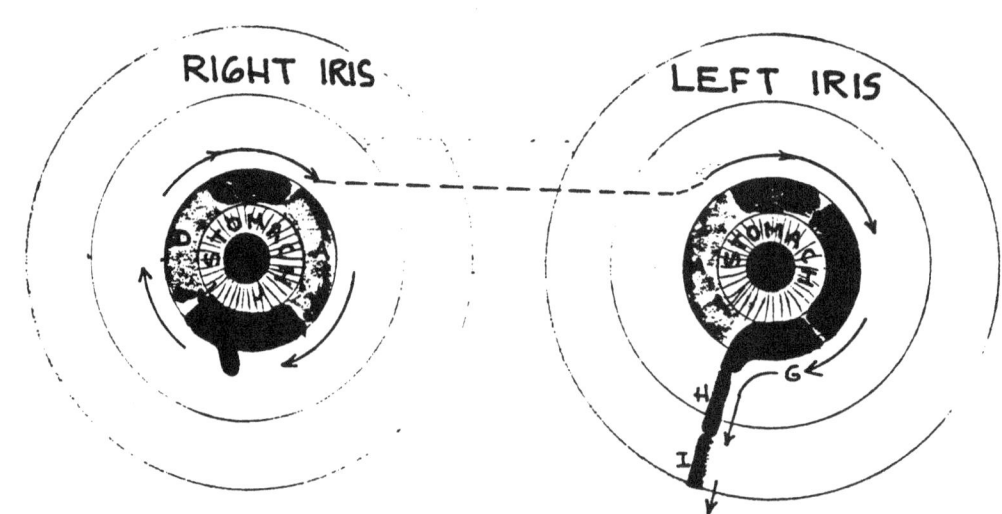

RIGHT IRIS   LEFT IRIS

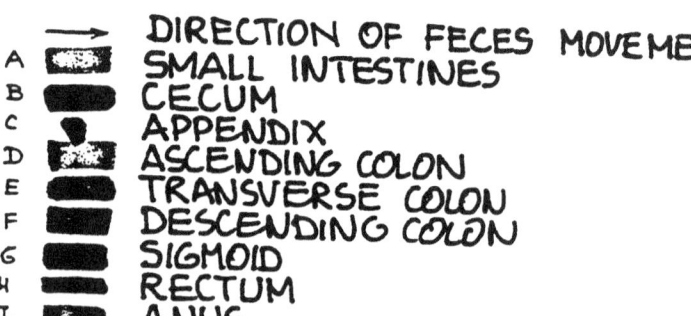

→ DIRECTION OF FECES MOVEMENT

A   SMALL INTESTINES
B   CECUM
C   APPENDIX
D   ASCENDING COLON
E   TRANSVERSE COLON
F   DESCENDING COLON
G   SIGMOID
H   RECTUM
I   ANUS

O BOWELS CONDITIONS

A — DARK BROWN BOWELS RING:
 INDICATES: CONSTIPATION

B — STRICTURE:
 INDICATES: SPASM IN BOWELS
 MUSCLES, NARROWING IN SOME
 PARTS OF LARGE INTESTINE
 AND DETERIORATED PARISTALTIC
 WAVE. CONSTIPATION.

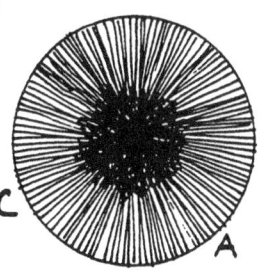
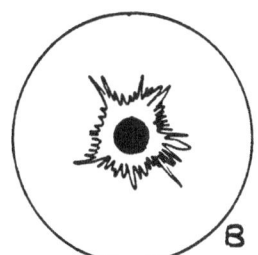

C — BALLOONED BOWEL:
 INDICATES: ENLARGED DESCENDING
 AND SIGMOID COLONS, COLITIS
 AND CONSTIPATION.

D — BOWEL POCKETS:
 INDICATES: FORMATION OF
 POCKETS OPENED FROM COLON
 WALL. CONSTIPATION, COLITIS.

E — DARK BOWEL POCKETS:
 INDICATES: CHRONIC
 DIVERTICULITIS, COLITIS
 AND CHRONIC CONSTIPATION.

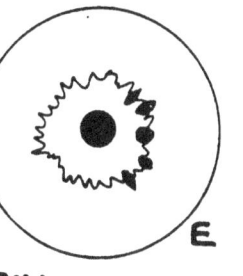
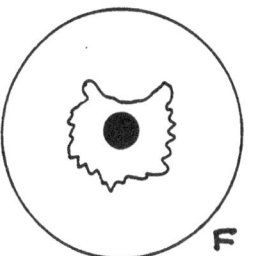

F — DECREASED UPPER SPACE
 BETWEEN ANW AND PUPIL:
 INDICATES: PROLAPSUS OF THE
 TRANSVERSE COLON.

G — VERY DARK CECUM:
 INDICATES: FECES ACCUMULATION
 AND CHRONIC CONSTIPATION
 CAUSED BY APPENDECTOMY.

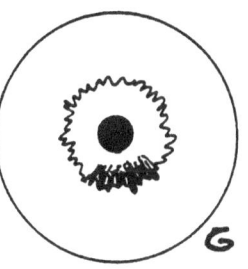
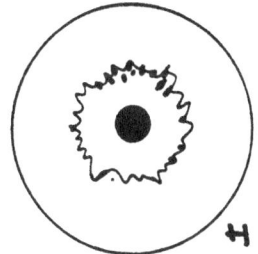

H — SMALL BLACK SPOTS IN ANW RIM:
 INDICATE: INTESTINAL
 PARASITIS

I — RADII SOLARIS:
 INDICATES: TOXIC SEEPAGE
 THROUGH INTESTINAL WALL
 VIA THE BLOOD STREAM
 INTO VARIOUS BODY ORGANS
 CAUSING SERIOUS ORGANS
 MALFUNCTION.

J — SMALL BLACK SPOTS IN ANUS
 AREA:
 INDICATES:
 HAEMORRHOIDS (PILES)
 CHRONIC CONSTIPATION.

CAUSES & TREATMENT:
 (SEE CONSTIPATION)

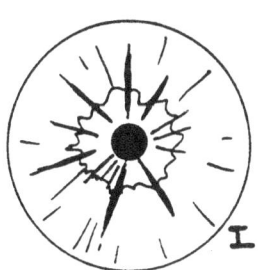
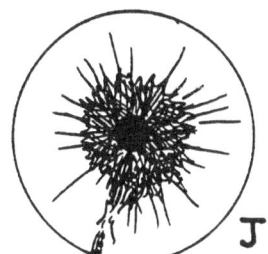

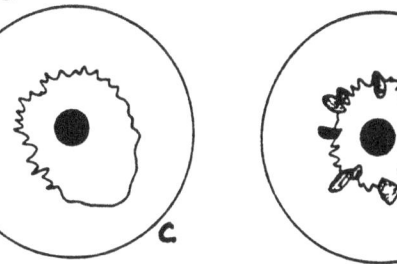

O BRAIN AREA'S CHART

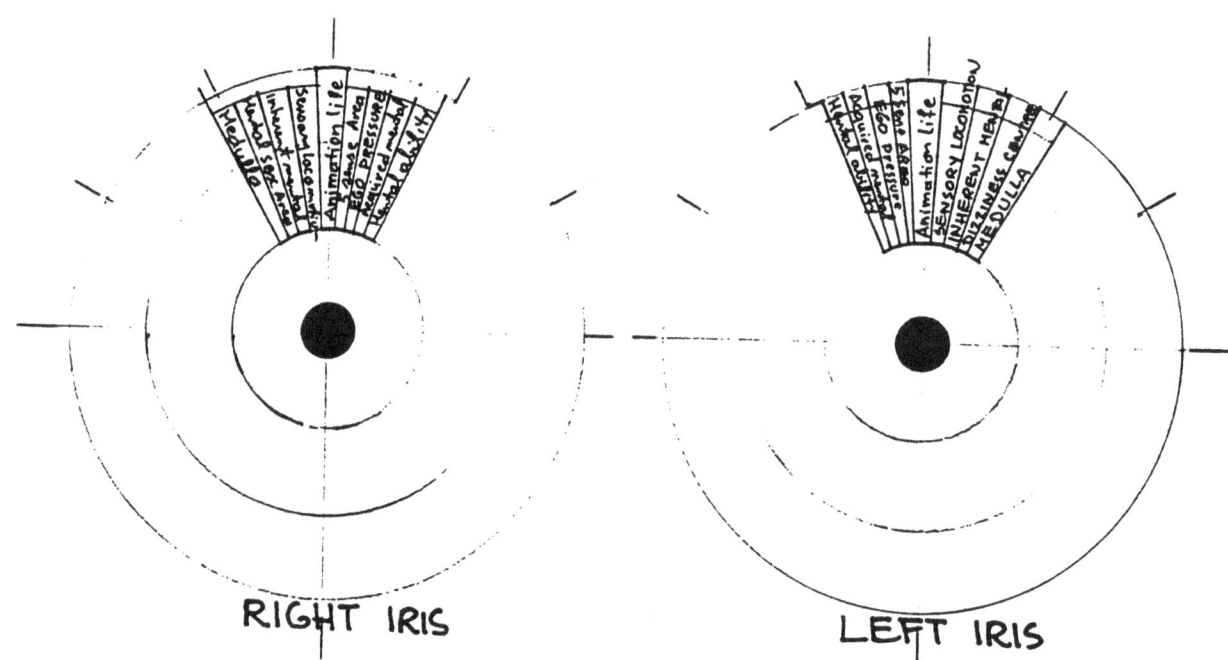

RIGHT IRIS   LEFT IRIS

O BRAIN CONDITIONS:

A — GOOD VITALITY, HIGH ENERGY:
WHITE SIGN IN ANIMATION
LIFE AREA.

B — PERMANENT LOSS OF
VITALITY:
DARK SIGN IN ANIMATION
LIFE AREA

C — ANXIETY:
BROWN SIGN IN INHERENT
MENTAL AREA, NERVE RINGS.

D — INSOMNIA:
WHITE SIGNS IN INHERENT
MENTAL AREA, COLOURED
ADRENAL GLAND, NERVERINGS

E — HYPER ACTIVITY:
WHITE SIGNS IN SENSORY
LOCOMOTION AREA.
WHITE NERVE RINGS.

F — FRUSTRATION & DIS-
SATISFACTION:
DARK SIGN IN MENTAL
ABILITY AREA, ZIG ZAG
FIBRES.

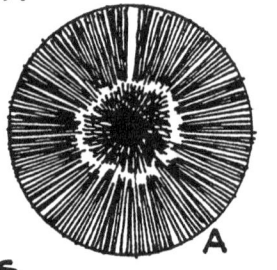
A

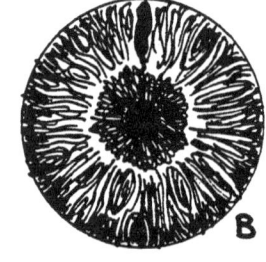
B

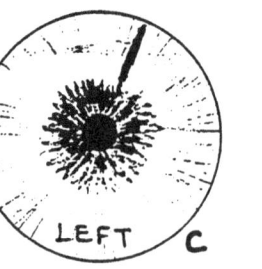
LEFT C

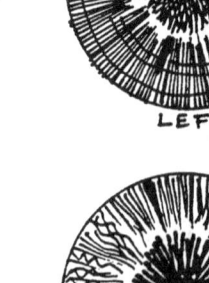
LEFT D

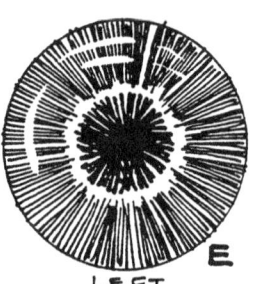
LEFT E

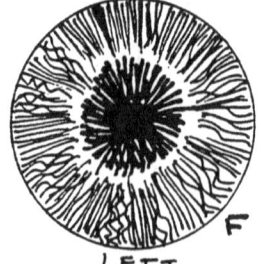
LEFT F

BRAIN CONDITIONS

G_ POOR MEMORY, TIREDNESS
LACK OF CONCENTRATION:
SODIUM RING PASSING
THROUGH BRAIN AREA.

H_ HYSTERIA:
WHITE NERVE RINGS
IN BRAIN AREA.

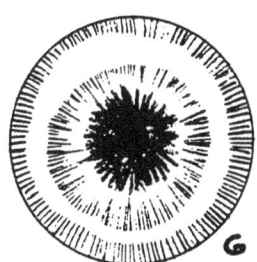
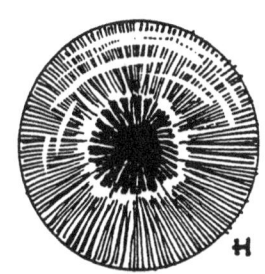

I_ DEPRESSION & EXHAUSTION
DARK BRAIN AREA
DARK ADRENAL GLAND
DARK THYROID GLAND

J_ MEMORY LOSS, PROSTATION
NUMBNESS, PARTIAL PARALYSIS
OF MENTAL AND NERVOUS
FUNCTIONS:
BLACK NERVE RINGS IN
BRAIN AREA

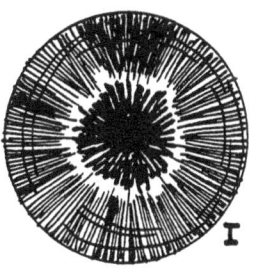
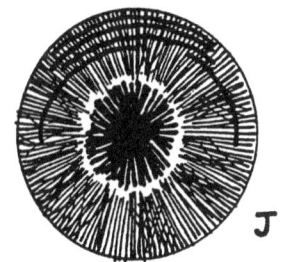

CAUSES: SEE NERVOUS SYSTEM
TREATMENT: SEE NERVOUS SYSTEM

O BREAST (SEE MAMMARY GLANDS)

O BRONCHIALS (SEE CHART PAGE B13)

O BRONCHUS (SEE CHART PAGE B13)

O BRONCHITIS

IRIS SIGNS:

A_ RAISED WHITE FIBRES IN LUNGS
AREA, DARK MEDULLA.
INDICATE: ACUTE STAGE OF
BRONCHITIS.

B_ BROWN WEAKNESS LESION
IN LEFT LOBE OF LUNG AREA.
INDICATES: A SUB ACUTE
STAGE OF BRONCHITIS.

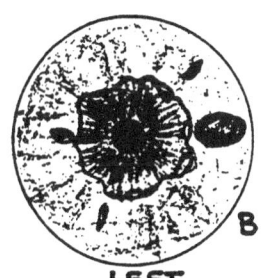

RIGHT   LEFT

C_ DARKNESS IN THE RIGHT LOBE
LUNGS EXTENDED INTO SCLERA.
DARK SCURF RIM & LYMPHIC
SIGNS. DARK MEDULLA.
INDICATE: CHRONIC BRONCHITIS
CONDITION

D_ RADII SOLERIS IN LUNGS
HEART, MEDULLA AND BRAIN.
NERVE RINGS, SCURF RIM
AND BLUE ANEMIA RING.
INDICATE: A VERY SERIOUS
CONDITION OF BRONCHITIS DEGENERATIVE STAGE.
CAUSING POOR & TOXIC CIRCULATION.

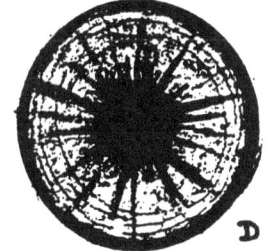

BRONCHITIS

CAUSES:

A. ACUTE STAGE.

ACIDITY
CATARRHAL SETTLEMENTS
EXCESS MUCUS FORMATION
POOR ELIMINATION
POOR RESPIRATION, POOR CIRCULATION.
CONSTIPATION
ANIMAL PROTEIN EXCESS
REFINED CARBOHYDRATES
DAIRY PRODUCTS
CITRUS FRUITS JUICE EXCESS
FIBRE DEFICIENCY
ALKALINE FOOD DEFICIENCY
A VITAMIN DEFICIENCY
ZINC DEFICIENCY
FRESH RAW FRUITS & VEGETABLES DEFICIENCY.
POOR BODY CONSTITUTION
MEDULLA WEAKNESS
POSTURE POOR ALIGNMENT
LACK OF PHYSICAL EXERCISE.

B. CHRONIC STAGE.

ACUTE BRONCHITIS
SUPPRESSED TREATMENT
PROLONGED DRUGS & ANTIBIOTIC THERAPY
CHRONIC CONSTIPATION
ANEMIA, POOR ASSIMILATION.
PERMANENT POLLUTED OCCUPATION
INTESTINAL PARASITIS (ASCARIS WORMS)
STRESS, ENDOCRINE IMBALANCES.
POOR CIRCULATION, TOXIC BLOOD
LYMPH CONGESTION.

WHOLISTIC RELATIONSHIPS:

RESPIRATORY & CIRCULATORY SYSTEMS.
RESPIRATORY & DIGESTIVE SYSTEMS
RESPIRATORY & NERVOUS SYSTEMS
RESPIRATORY & ENDOCRINE SYSTEMS.

TREATMENT:

BOWELS CLEANSING
VEGETABLE JUICE FASTING
POTASSIUM BROTH FASTING
ANTIBIOTICS NATURALLY (FD), PROPOLIS
ANEMIA FORMULA (FD), ASTHMA FORMULA (FD)
BLOOD CIRCULATION (FD) ALKALINE FORMULA (FD)
BLOOD PURIFYING (Dr.C)
ENHANCE MEDULLA FUNCTION, ALEXANDER TECHNIQUE
CHIROPRACTICE.
CASTOR OIL PACKS

NOTE: ELIMINATING WORMS SHOULD START BEFORE ANY
FASTING PROGRAME.

* CHART TO IRIDOLOGY

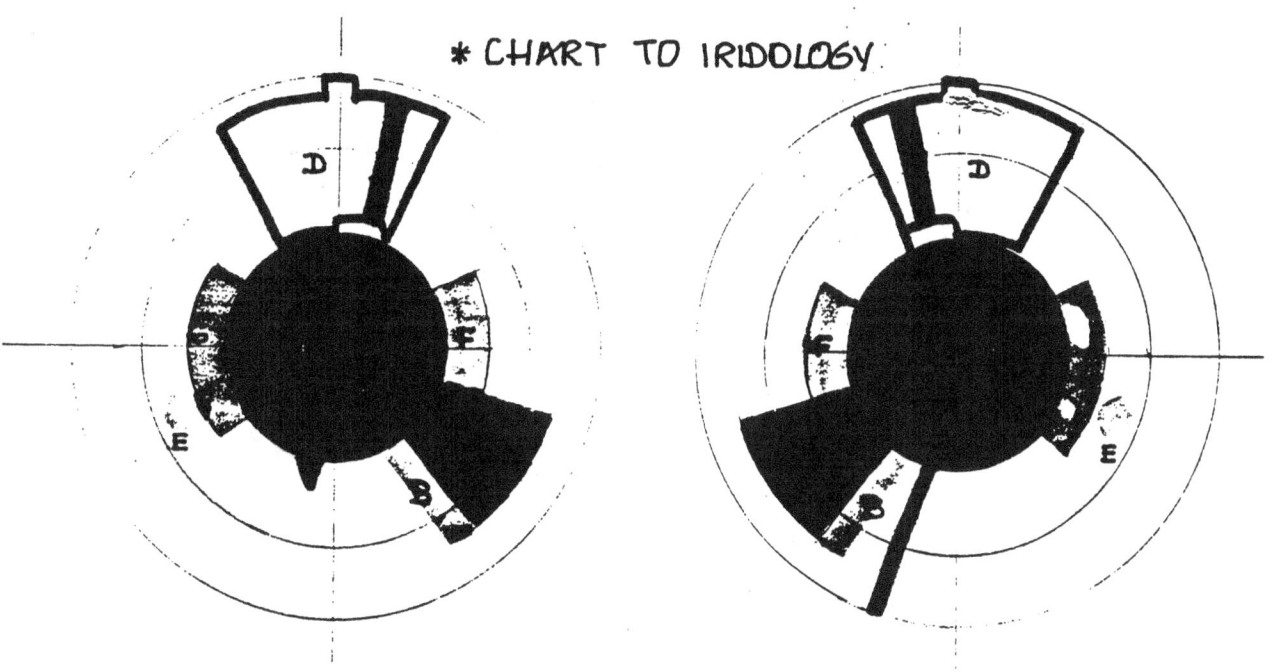

- ◼ BACK AREA
- ◼ BLADDER
- BONE AREA (SEE SKELETAL SYSTEM)
- ◼ BOWELS AREA (SEE DETAILS PAGE B8)
- ▥ BRAIN AREA (SEE DETAILS PAGE B10)
- ▤ BREAST (MAMMARY GLANDS)
- ▥ BRONCHUS
- ◼ BRONCHIALS
- ◼ BLOOD PRESSURE AREA

* BASED ON CHARTS TO IRIDOLOGY DEVELOPED BY
  Dr. BERNARD JENSEN AND DOROTHY HALL

○ CALCIUM DEFICIENCY

IRIS SIGNS:

A — *HESSIAN TYPE STRUCTURE
OR *DENSITY 5-6
OR WEEK CONSTITUTION.
IRIS REVEALS A CONDITION
OF CALCIUM DEFICIENCY
OR CALCIUM POOR RESERVE.
A PERMANENT CALCIUM
AWARENESS IS RECOMMENDED.

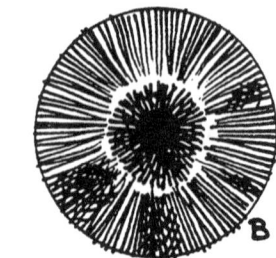

B — LEFT IRIS: DARKNESS IN
BONE AREAS, BACK NECK
SHOUDER & HAND & LEG
INDICATE: POOR POSTURE
AND CALCIUM DEFICIENCY

C — CHRONIC CONSTIPATION
AND LYMPHATIC CONGESTION
INDICATE: CALCIUM, MAGNESIUM
& POTASSIUM DEFICIENCY

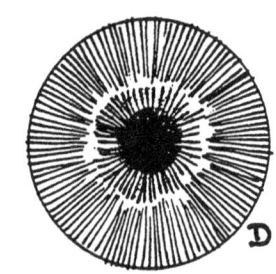

D — UNDER ACID STOMACH, HYDROCHLORIC ACID DEFICIENCY
INDICATE POOR CALCIUM ABSORBTION & CALCIUM DEFICIENCY.

○ CALCIUM IMBALANCE

IRIS SIGNS:

E — SODIUM RING
INDICATES: FAULTY DIET
OF CALCIUM & SODIUM
SOURCES.
CALCIUM DEPOSIT IN
ARTERY WALLS, CALCIUM
SODIUM IMBALANCE.

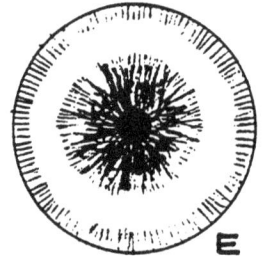
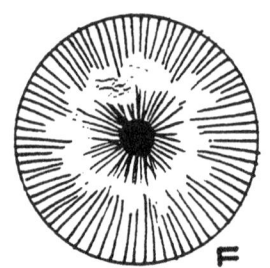

F — RAISED WHITE FIBRES
INDICATE: CALCIUM, PHOSPHOROUS
MAGNESIUM IMBALANCE.

G — PARATHYROID & THYROID
MALFUNCTION
INDICATE: POOR CALCIUM
METABOLISM

H — PROLAPSUS OF THE
TRANSVERSE COLON
INDICATE: CALCIUM
IMBALANCE AND DEFICIENCY.

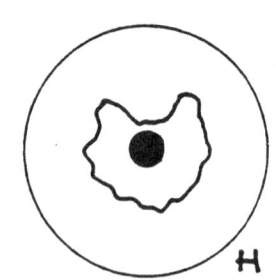

CAUSES & TREATMENT:
SEE SKELETAL SYSTEM.

* "HESSIAN TYPE" IRIS AS DESCRIBED BY DOROTHY HALL.
"DENSITY" AS DESCRIBED BY Dr. BERNARD JENSEN

O CANCER

IRIS SIGNS:

A _ BLACK LACUNE IN GALL BLADDER
AREA, BLACK NERVE RINGS
OVER LIVER AREA, DRUG SPOTS.
INDICATE:
A DEGENERATIVE GALL
STONES CONDITION
OR CANCER IN THE GALL_
BLADDER.

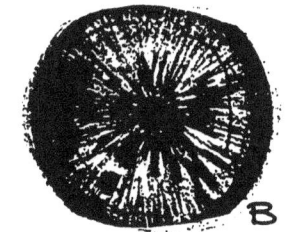

B _ BLACK THICK SCURF RIM
EXTENDED INTO LUNG AREA
BRAIN & LEGS ANEMEA DUE
TO REDUCED BLOOD CIRCULATION
INDICATE:
DEGENERATIVE LUNGS
CONDITION, TUBERCULOSIS
OR LUNG CANCER

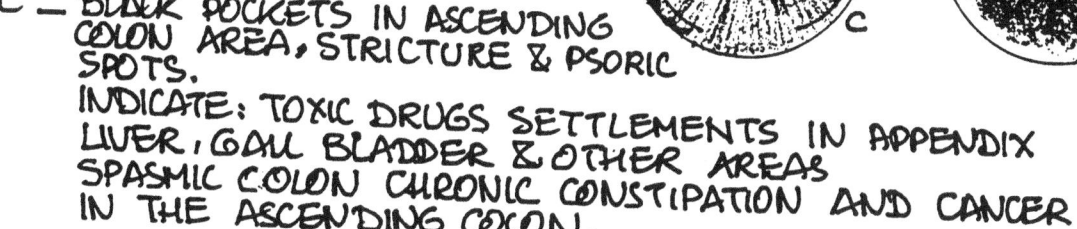

C _ BLACK POCKETS IN ASCENDING
COLON AREA, STRICTURE & PSORIC
SPOTS.
INDICATE: TOXIC DRUGS SETTLEMENTS IN APPENDIX
LIVER, GALL BLADDER & OTHER AREAS
SPASMIC COLON CHRONIC CONSTIPATION AND CANCER
IN THE ASCENDING COLON.

D _ THICK ANEMIA RING, DARK BOWELS, RADII SOLERIS.
INDICATES: DEGENERATIVE BOWELS CONDITION & ABSENT
FUNCTION OF THE SKIN & FINE CAPILLARIES
OR SKIN CANCER.

CAUSES:
ORTHODOX SUPPRESSED TREATMENTS FOR VARIOUS ORGANS
DISEASES, PROLONGED DRUGS CONSUMPTION.
UN-TREATED CHRONIC & DEGENERATIVE CONDITIONS.
OVER CONSUMPTION OF ANIMAL SOURCES FOODS, FATS EXCESS.
VEGETABLES & FRUITS DEFICIENCY.
A, C & E VITAMINES DEFICIENCY.
MINERAL IMBALANCES / SELENIUM DEFICIENCY.
POLLUTION, STRESS, FOOD ADDITIVES
POOR OXYGENATION
CONSTIPATION
ABSENT ELIMINATIVE FUNCTION & ABSENT NUTRIENT
ABSORBTION
LACK OF PHYSICAL EXERCISE & POOR VENTILATION
EMOTIONAL STRESS, FRUSTRATIONS.

WHOLISTIC RELATION SHIPS.
ALL SYSTEMS INVOLVED
TREATMENT:
GREEN LEAVES (BROTH & RAW) LONG FAST.
PLAIN WATER FAST.
REST, MEDITATION.

○ CAPILLARIES (SEE CIRCULATORY SYSTEM)

○ CATARACT (SEE EYE'S DISEASES)

○ CATARRH (SEE ALSO ACIDITY)

IRIS SIGNS:
WHITENESS

INDICATIONS:
EXCESS MUCUS FORMATION
ACIDIC CONDITION
TOXIC ACCUMULATION
ARTHRITIS, GOUT, BURSITIS

CAUSES:
POOR ELIMINATION, POOR DRAINAGE.
ACIDIC FOODS EXCESS
ALKALINE FOODS DEFICIENCY

WHOLISTIC RELATIONSHIPS:
(SEE ACIDITY)

TREATMENT:
(SEE ACIDITY & ARTHRITIS)

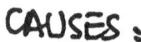

○ CECUM (SEE CHART PAGE B8)

○ CENTRAL NERVOUS SYSTEM CHARTS

IRIS SIGNS:

A _ CHART TO CNS

B _ HEALTHY CNS.
ZONE 1 PUPIL AND
STOMACH RING.

C _ UN HEALTHY CNS.
ZONE 1 PUPIL AND
STOMACH RING
(SEE ZONES)

D _ CEREBRAL WEAKNESS.
RADIALS FROM CNS
INTO BRAIN AREA.

E _ WEAK LEG MUSCLES.
RADIALS FROM CNS
INTO LEG AREA.

* THIS TYPE OF RADIALS
RADIATING FROM THE CNS
INDICATE ABNORMALITIES
IN THE ORGANS CONTROLLED
BY CEREBRAL & CEREB-
ELLUM FUNCTIONS, LIKE
MUSCLES & FIVE SENSES.

○ CERVIX
(SEE CHART PAGE C12)

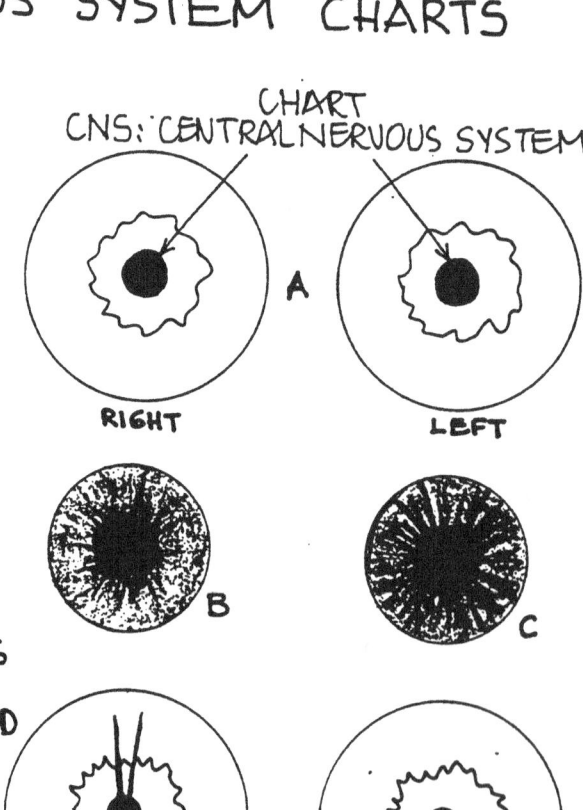

CHART
CNS: CENTRAL NERVOUS SYSTEM

RIGHT   LEFT

A

B   C

D   E

O CHARTS TO IRIDOLOGY
DEVELOPED BY Dr. BERNARD JENSEN

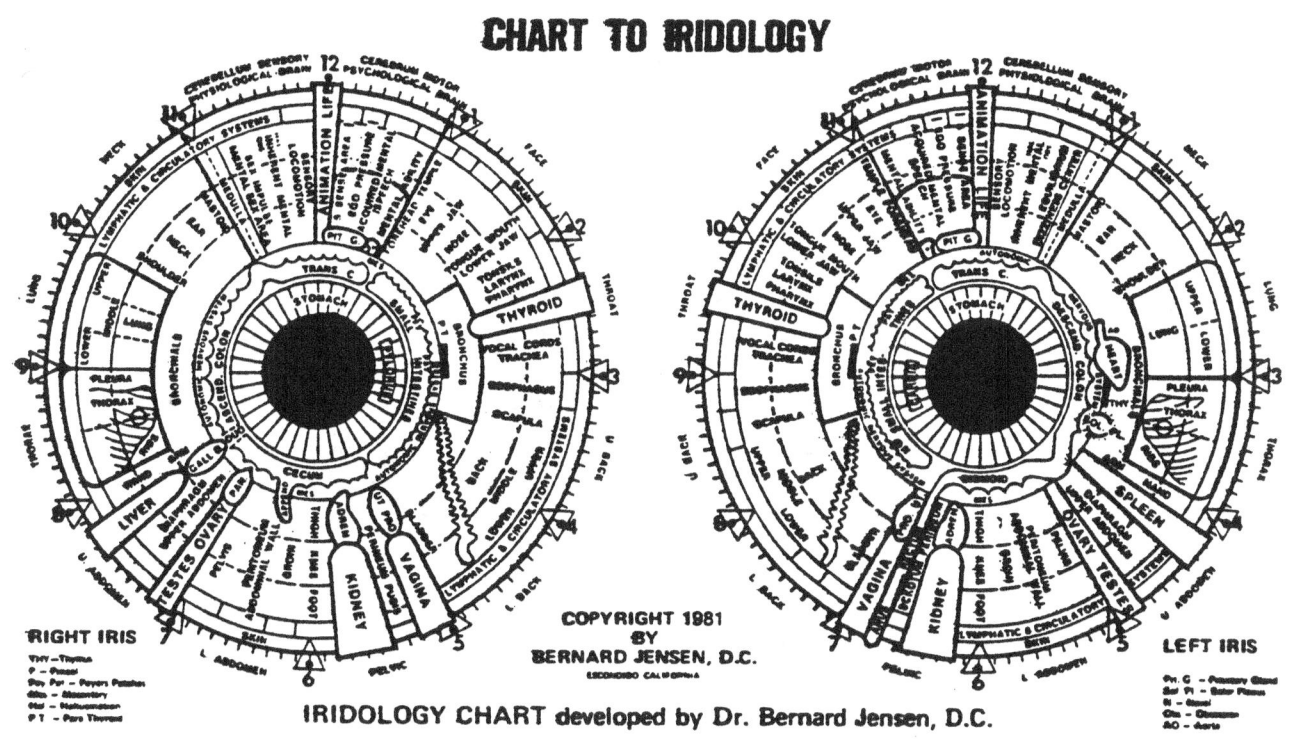

IRIDOLOGY CHART developed by Dr. Bernard Jensen, D.C.

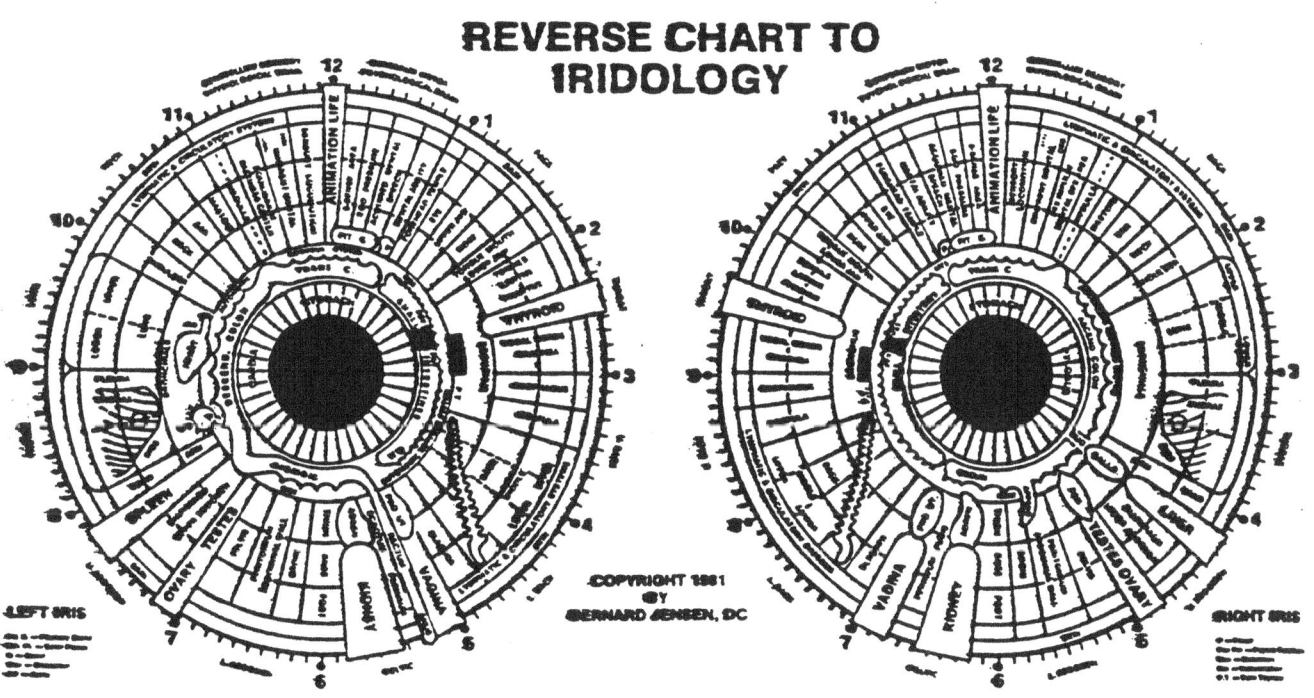

This reversed chart is to be used in self-analysis as it matches the reversed image of the eye as seen in a mirror.

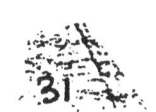

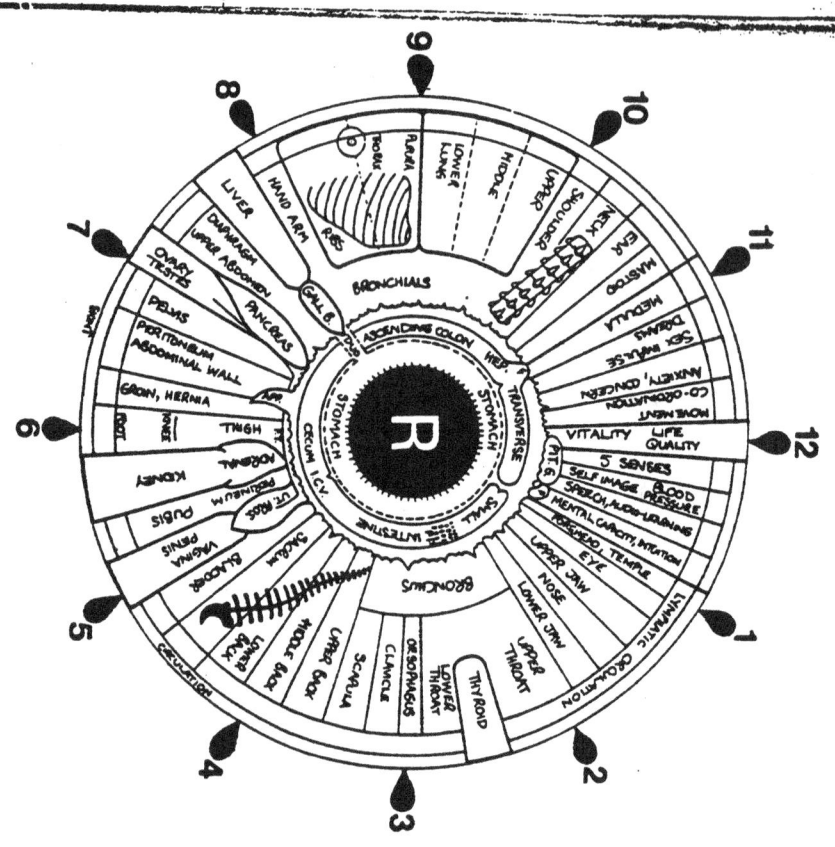

The Iris Map, right eye
(looking at another person's right eye)

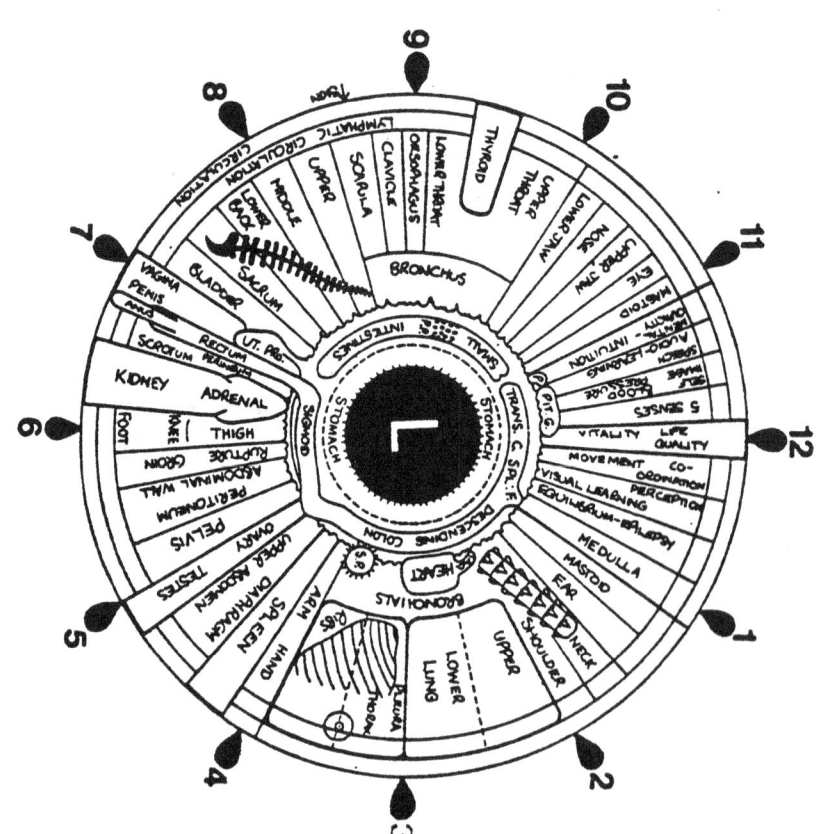

The Iris Map, left eye
(looking at another person's left eye)

O CHEST AREA (SEE CHART PAGE C12)

O CHOLESTEROL DEPOSITS
IRIS SIGNS:
SODIUM RING
INDICATIONS:
SODIUM, CALCIUM & CHOLESTEROL DEPOSITS.
CAUSES:
UN ORGANIC SODIUM EXCESS.
SATURATED FATS EXCESS.
REFINED CARBOHYDRATES EXCESS.
MINERALS IMBALANCE.
EMULSIFIERS DEFICIENCY
LECITHIN, E VITAMIN, C VITAMIN
PECTIN, GARLIC, ONION, CELERY.
SLOW BLOOD CIRCULATION, LACK OF PHYSICAL EXERCISE.
ALKALINE FOOD DEFICIENCY.
EMOTIONAL STRESS

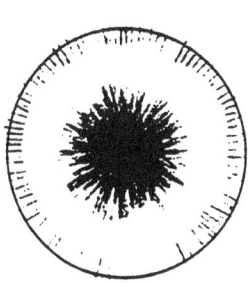

WHOLISTIC RELATION SHIPS:
CIRCULATORY & DIGESTIVE SYSTEMS
CIRCULATORY & MUSCULAR SYSTEMS
CIRCULATORY & ENDOCRINE SYSTEMS
CIRCULATORY & RESPIRATORY SYSTEMS

TREATMENT:
BOWELS CLEANSING
BLOOD PURIFICATION HERBAL FORMULA (PD)
BLOOD CIRCULATION (PD)
STRICT VEGAN DIET
LECITHIN
WHEAT GERM OIL
APPLE MONO DIET FASTING
FRESH RAW VEGETABLES JUICES.
PHYSICAL EXERCISE.

O CHRONIC STAGE OF DISEASE
IRIS SIGNS:
DARK GREY OR BROWN LESIONS IN ORGAN AREAS.
INDICATIONS: CHRONIC STAGE OF DISEASE.
CAUSES: FREQUENT ACUTE CASES
IGNORED WITHOUT TREATMENT.
ANTIBIOTIC SUPPRESSED TREATMENT.
ACUTE CAUSATIVE FACTORS
UNCHANGED FOR LONG PERIODS
OF TIME.
INHERITED WEAKNESSES.
DRUGS SETTLEMENTS.
WHOLISTIC RELATION SHIPS:
DEPENDS UPON THE ORGANS.
TREATMENT: (SEE STAGES OF DISEASE)

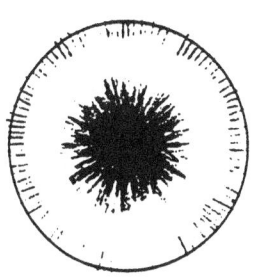

O CIRCULATORY SYSTEM CHART
(SEE ALSO CHART PAGE A14)

* CHART TO IRIDOLOGY

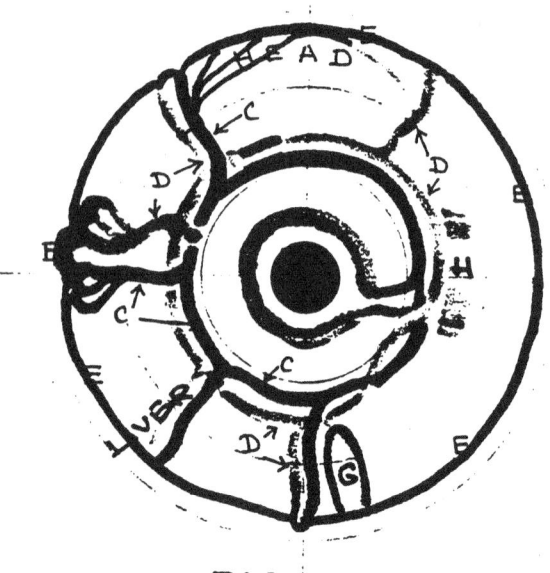
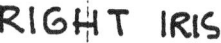
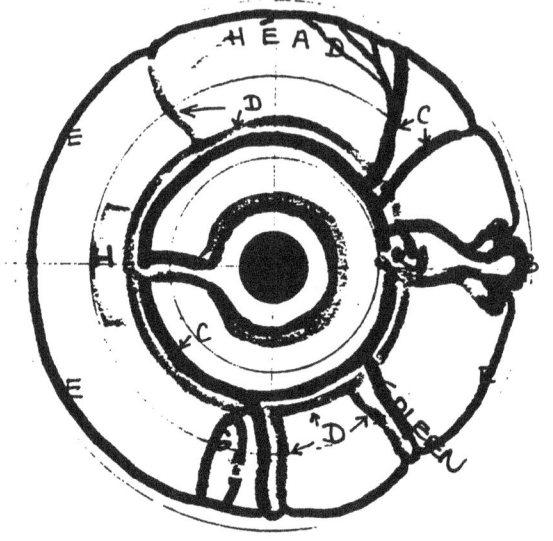

RIGHT IRIS   LEFT IRIS

- HEART
- ALVEOLIS (LUNGS)
- ARTERIES
- VEINS
- CAPILLARIES
- GASTRIC CIRCULATION
- KIDNEYS
- BRONCHUS

* BASED ON FUNDAMENTAL BASIS OF IRISDIAGNOSIS BY THEODOR KRIEGE.

O CIRCULATORY SYSTEM DISEASES.

IRIS SIGNS:

A_ ANEMIA AT BRAIN
AND EXTREMETIES
(SEE PAGE A5)

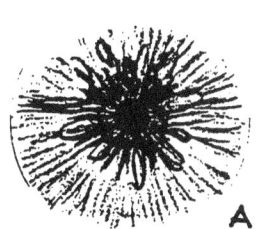
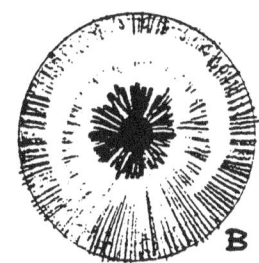

B_ SODIUM RING
INDICATES:
HARDNING OF ARTERIES
CHOLESTEROLE DEPOSITS.

C_ SCURF RIM
INDICATES:
POOR BLOOD SUPPLY INTO
CADILLARIES & UNDERACTIVE
SKIN.
THE DARKER THE THICKER
THE MORE SERIOUS THE
DISEASE.

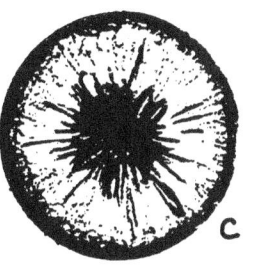
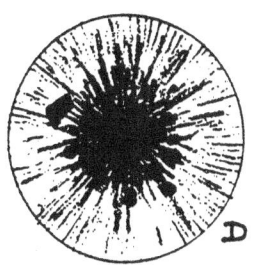

D_ TOXIC CIRCULATION
INDICATED BY ANW
DISCOLOURATIONS. AND
PSORIC SPOTS.

E_ TOXIC CIRCULATION
AND SINUSITIS INDICATED
BY DISCOLORATION EXTENDED
FROM ANW INTO HEAD AREA.

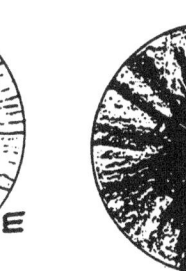

F_ TOXIN OVER LOAD FROM
CONSTIPATION CONDITION
THREATENS HEART, KIDNEYS.
INDICATED BY DARK BOWELS
AREA & RADII SOLERIS.

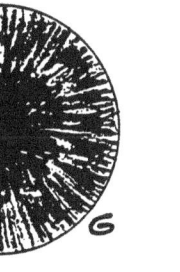
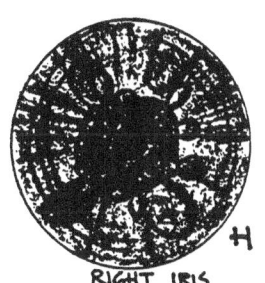

G_ HEAVY BURDEN OF TOXINS
IN CIRCULATORY SYSTEM
INDICATED BY CHRONIC
LYMPH CONGESTION & DARK
BOWEL AREA.

H_ OVER STRESSED LIVER
CAUSING POOR BLOOD
NOURISHMENT. INDICATED BY
WEAKNESS LESION & NERVE
RINGS IN LIVER AREA.

RIGHT IRIS

I_ POOR RESPIRATION & BLOOD SHORT
OXYGENATION. INDICATED BY
WEAKNESS LESION IN MEDULLA
AND LUNGS AREAS.

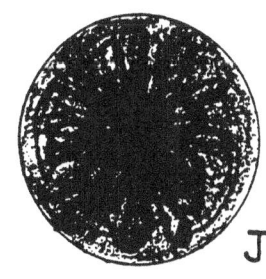

J_ POOR BLOOD CIRCULATION
POOR NUTRIENT ASSIMILATION
CAUSED BY CONSTIPATION
BOWELS POCKETS AND
INTESTINAL PARASITIS
INDICATED BY: POOR
CONSTITUTION, DARK BOWEL AREA
BLACK CRYPTS IN ANW, BOWEL POCKETS
WEAKNESS LESIONS, LACK OF TONE.
SPINAL LESIONS, POOR POSTURE

CIRCULATORY SYSTEM DISEASES.
CAUSES:
     ANIMAL FATS EXCESS
     ANIMAL SOURCES PROTEIN
     DAIRY PRODUCTS
     REFINED CARBOHYDRATES
     ACID ALKALINE IMBALANCE
     TEA, COFFE, ALCOHOLS, DRUGS, SMOCKINGS
     SEX EXCESS
     REST EXCESS
     FIBRE DEFICIENCY
     FRESH FRUITS & VEGETABLES DEFICIENCY
     RAW VEGETABLES DEFICIENCY
     ANTI THROMBUS & EMULSIFIERS DEFICIENCY
        LECITHINE, POLYUNSATURATED FATY ACIDS
        E & C VITAMINS.
     LACK OF PHYSICAL EXERCISE
     EMOTIONAL STRESS
     INHERITED WEAKNESS WITH INHERITED LIFE STYLE.
     MODERN CIVILIZATION
     PULLUTION
     POOR BREATHING HABITS
     LACK OF PROPER VENTILATION
     CONSTIPATION
     LIVER WEAKNESS UN ABLE TO CLEAN BLOOD
     KIDNEY WEAKNESS
     MUDULLA OBLANGATA WEAKNESS
     THORACIC LESIONS
     POOR POSTURE, POOR CONSTITUTION.
     LYMPH CONGESTION
     ANEMEIC CONDITIONS.
     ENDOCRINE IMBALANCES.
WHOLISTIC RELATIONSHIPS.
     CIRCULATORY SYSTEM AND ALL SYSTEMS

TREATMENT:
     BLOOD CIRCULATION A (DrC), BLOOD PURIFYING (DrC).
     BLOOD CIRCULATION B (FD).
     ANEMIA FORMULA (FD)/LYMPHATIC FORMULA (FD).
     BOWELS CLEANSING.
     LIVER FLUSH/GALL BLADDER CLEANS/CASTOR OIL PACKS.
     ORGANIC IRON SOURCES WITH C VITAMIN.
     MULTI MINERAL & VITAMINS NATURALLY (FD).
     LECITHIN, E VITAMIN, IRON, MAGNESIUM, CALCIUM
        IODINE, CHLORINE, PHOSPHOROUS FROM VEGETARIAN
     ORGANICALLY GROWN SOURCES.
     BREATHING EXERCISE.
     PHYSICAL EXERCISE.
     VEGETABLES JUICES.
     FOR HEART DISEASE, CORONARY ARTERIES, THROMBOSIS
        CHOLESTEROLE DEPOSITS, ARTERIOSCLEROSIS, URIC ACID
        A STRICT VEGAN DIET IS RECOMMENDED.

O COCCYX (SEE CHART PAGE C12)

O COLITIS (SEE CONSTIPATION)

O COLON (SEE BOWELS CHART PAGE B8)

O CONSTIPATION

IRIS SIGNS:

A_ HESSIEN TYPE, WEAK CONSTITUTION LACK OF TONE. INDICATE: A BODY PRONE TO DIGESTIVE DISORDERS & CONSTIPATION.

B_ NO FIBRES VISIBLE, BROWN IRIS. INDICATE: A BODY PRONE TO CONSTIPATION, KIDNEY DISEASE AND FLATULENCE.

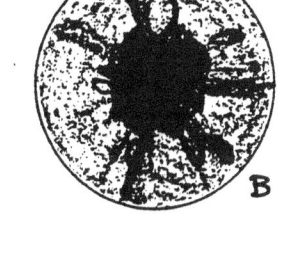

C_ DARK BOWEL AREA. INDICATE CONSTIPATION

D_ DARK BOWEL AREA WITH DISCOLORATION OUTSIDE ANW. INDICATE CHRONIC CONSTIPATION & TOXIN LADENED INTESTINES.

E_ BROWN FLARES IN CECUM AND EGO PRESSURE AREAS INDICATE: WEAK PARISTALSIS MUSCLES & STRESS. APPENDIX TROUBLE, CONSTIPATION & FLATULENCE.

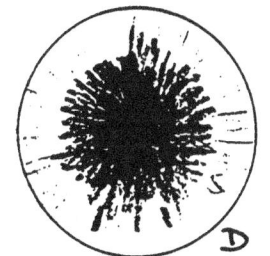

F_ STRICTURE ANW. INDICATE: SPASM OF COLON'S MUSCLES DUE TO DEGENERATIVE CONSTIPATION CONDITION.

G_ DARK BROWN LESIONS INSIDE ANW INDICATE: CHRONIC CONSTIPATION TOXIN LADENED BOWEL POCKETS DIVERTICULAE. VERY SMALL BLACK SPOTS INDICATE PARASITIS.

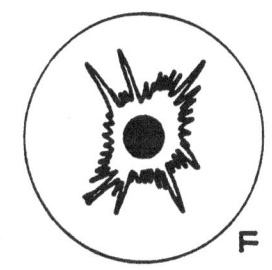

H_ VERY DARK BOWEL AREA RADII SOLERIS & NERVE RINGS INDICATE: CHRONIC CONSTIPATION TOXINS SEEPAGE INTO BODY ORGANS/SEVER IRRITATION IN THE INTESTINAL WALLS AND POSSIBILITY OF BLEEDING INTESTINE

I_ DILATED ANW LEFT IRIS IN DESCENDING COLON AREA INDICATE: BALLOONED BOWEL AT DESCENDING & SIGMOID COLONS COLITIS, PAIN, CHRONIC CONSTIPATION & FLATULENCE.

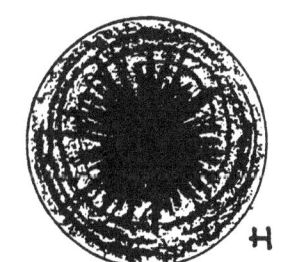

J_ CLEAR LIGHT BROWN, LESS CONTRAST COLOUR, WHITE FIBRES FILLING LESIONS. INDICATE HEALING SIGNS AFTER AN

* ULTIMATE BOWELS CLEANSING PROGRAM.

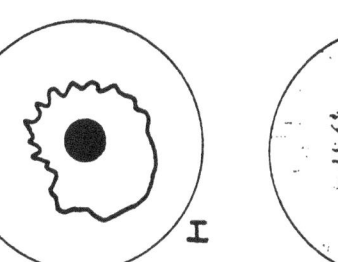

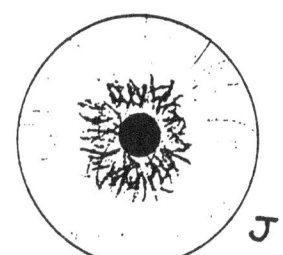

* REFERED TO TISSUE CLEANSING THROUGH BOWEL MANAGEMENT BY Dr. BERNARD JENSEN.

CONSTIPATION.
CAUSES:
REFINED CARBOHYDRATES
MEAT, FISH, EGGS DAIRY EXCESS
MIXING WHITE BREAD WITH CHEESE
PIZZA
FIBRE DEFICIENCY
FRESH RAN FRUITS DEFICIENCY
FRESH RAN VEGETABLES DEFICIENCY
POOR CHEWING
OVER BOILED FOODS, FRIED FOODS
POLISHED RICE
SEDENTARY OCCUPATION
LACK OF PHYSICAL EXERCISE
LACK OF EXPOSING THE BODY TO FRESH COLD AIR
LIVER UNDER FUNCTION
LACK OF FLUIDS
INHERITED WEAK BODY TONE, WEAK CONSTITUTION
MODERN CIVILIZATION
STRESS, PHYSICAL & EMOTIONAL
APPENDECTOMY.
ENDOCRINE IMBALANCE.

WHOLISTIC RELATION SHIPS.
DIGESTIVE & MUSCULAR SYSTEMS
DIGESTIVE & ENDOCRINE SYSTEMS
DIGESTIVE & URINARY SYSTEMS
DIGESTIVE & CIRCULATORY SYSTEMS

TREATMENT:
BOWEL CLEANSING, ENEMAS.
LIVER FLUSHING, GALL BLADDER CLEANS.
CASTOR OIL PACKS ON ABDOMINAL AREA.
FRESH RAN VEGETABLE JUICE FASTING. OR FRUITS.
    CARROTS, APPLES, GRAPES, WATER MELLON
COLITIS FORMULA (FD)
RECTAL BOLUS (FD)
POTASSIUM BROTH
HONEY APPLE CIDER VINAGAR DRINK.
PREVENTIVE DIET:
WHOLE WHEAT WITH BRAN.
FRESH RAN VEGETABLES MAIN MEALS
NUTS, RAISINS, DATES, DRIED FIGS
WHOLE RICE, MUSLI, WHEAT GERM.
LEAN MEATS NOT MORE THAN 4 TIMES MONTHLY
    WITH LEAFY VEGETABLES.
DRIED FRUITS BROTH
CAROB BROTH
PHYSICAL EXERCISE, SWIMMING.
EXPOSING BODY TO NATURAL CLIMATE CONDITIONS
FRESH AIR BATHING
SUN BATHING.
WARM & COLD WATER SHOWERS.

O CYSTITIS (SEE BLADDER DISEASE)

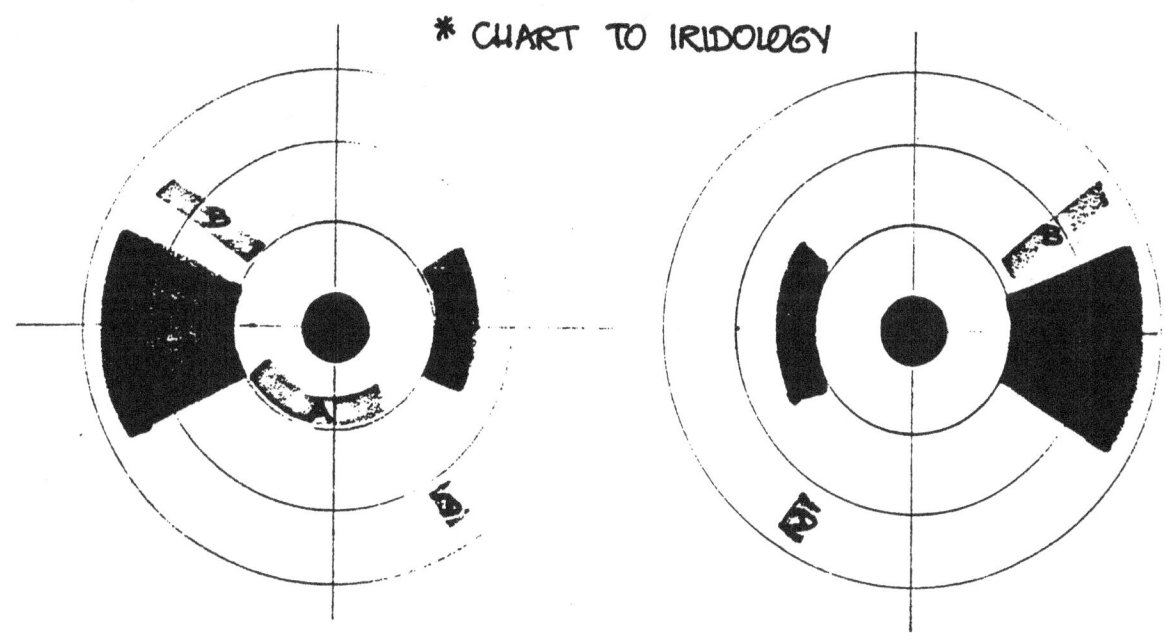

* CHART TO IRIDOLOGY

[A] CECUM
[B] CERVIX
[C] CHEST ZONES
[D] COCCYX

* BASED ON CHARTS TO IRIDOLOGY DEVELOPED BY
Dr. BERNARD JENSEN AND DOROTHY HALL

O DARK IRIS

IRIS SIGNS:

BROWN IRIS (USUALLY)
DARK BROWN IRIS COLOUR
INDICATES: CHRONIC TOXIC
ACCUMULATIONS, CONSTIPATION
CATARRH, SLUGGISH LYMPH
AND BLOOD CIRCULATIONS.

CAUSES: BROWN IRIS TYPE
ABDOMINAL DISORDERS.
VERY POOR ELIMINATIVE
CHANNELS: SKIN, KIDNEYS
BOWELS, LUNGS.
POOR CONSITUTION.
LACK OF PHYSICAL ACTIVITY.

WHOLISTIC RELATION SHIPS:
DIGESTIVE & CIRCULATORY SYSTEMS
DIGESTIVE & URINARY SYSTEMS.
DIGESTIVE & RESPIRATORY SYSTEMS
DIGESTIVE & ENDOCRINE SYSTEMS.

TREATMENT:
BOWELS CLEANSING
LIVER FLUSH & GALL BLADDER CLEANSING
CASTOR OIL ABDOMINAL PACKS
BLOOD PURIFICATION (FD)
KIDNEYS CLEANSING.
MONO DIETS FAST
PHYSICAL EXERCISE
CVITAMIN & IRON NATURALY.

O DEAFNESS

IRIS SIGNS:

A— DARK EAR AREA, NERVE RINGS
DARK RADII SOLERIS RADIATING
FROM CNS.
DARK 5 SENSE AREA IF THE
CONDITIONS CAUSED BY CEREBRAL
WEAKNESS.

B— WHITE RAISED FIBERS IN THE
5 SENSE AREA (IF THE CONDITION
OF DEAFNESS IS INHERITED OR
CAUSED BY SEVER CHRONIC EAR
INFECTION) AS AN INDICATION OF
OVER ACTIVITY OF THE OTHER
SENSES. TO BALANCE THE HEARING
WEAKNESS.
FRUSTRATION SIGNS & NERVE RINGS
MAY EXIST.

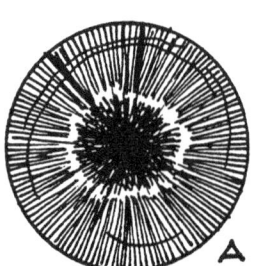

A

RIGHT

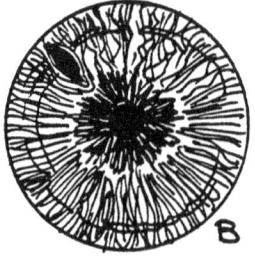

B

RIGHT

CAUSES:
INHERITED WEAKNESSES
UNTREATED INFECTIONS.
INFECTIONS TREATMENTS BY ORTHODOX
SUPPRESSIVE DRUGS.
VERY NOISY OCCUPATION, CONSTRUCTION
EQUIPMENT, GENERATORS, ECT.

DEAFNESS
CAUSES
DEGENERATIVE DISEASES.
CERVICAL LESIONS.
TRAUMA
ACCIDENTS, INJURY

WHOLISTIC RELATION SHIPS:

NERVOUS & CIRCULATORY SYSTEMS
NERVOUS & LYMPHIC SYSTEMS
NERVOUS & ENDOCRINE SYSTEMS

O DEGENERATIVE STAGE OF DISEASE

IRIS SIGNS:
DARKNES IN ORGAN AREA
DARKNES IN ORGANS WITH RELATION
SHIPS.
INDICATIONS:
CHRONIC & DEGENERATIVE STAGE
IN THE ORGANIS AREA.

A _ TUBERCULOSIS

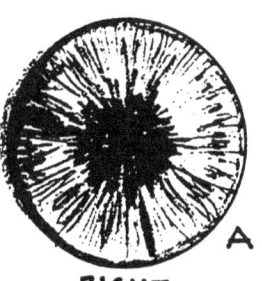
RIGHT

B _ HYPOTHYROIDISM
(SEE HYPER & HYPOTHYROIDISM, THYROID PAGE   )

C _ KIDNEY FAILURE.
(SEE KIDNEY DISEASE PAGE   )

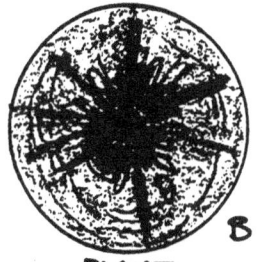
RIGHT

CAUSES,
POOR CONSTITUTION
PROLONGED DRUGS THERAPY
SUPPRESSED ACUTE STAGES
POOR ELIMINATION
CONSTIPATION
DIETERY FAULTY HABITS

WHOLISTIC RELATION SHIPS:
ALL SYSTEMS INVOLVED

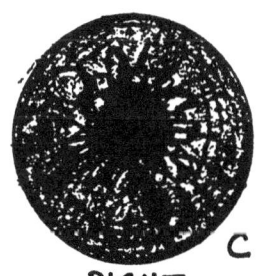
RIGHT

TREATMENT:
ULTIMATE BOWELS CLEANSING (Dr. BJ)
LIVER FLUSHING GALL BLADDER CLEANSE
STIMULATE ALL ELIMINATIVE CHANNELS
WATER FASTING
HERBS FASTINGS
BLOOD PURIFICATION (FD)
BLOOD CIRCULATION (FD & DrC)
MEDITATION
REST.

O DEPRESSION

IRIS SIGNS:

A_ DEPRESSION CAUSED BY
   NERVOUS IRRITATIONS
   INDICATED BY BLACK LESIONS
   IN BRAIN AREA

B_ DEPRESSION CAUSED BY
   ENDOCRINE IMBALACES
   INDICATED BY DISCOLORATIONS
   IN GLANDS AREAS.

C_ DEPRESSION CAUSED BY
   HYPOGLYCEMIA
   INDICATED BY DISCOLORATIONS
   IN PANCREAS & BOWELS
   AREAS.

D_ DEPRESSION CAUSED BY
   FAILURE AND FRUSTRATIONS
   INDICATED BY DILATED PUPIL
   RAISED WHITE ZIGZAG FIBERS.

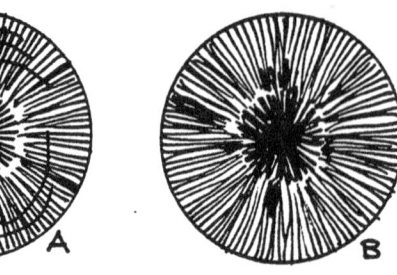

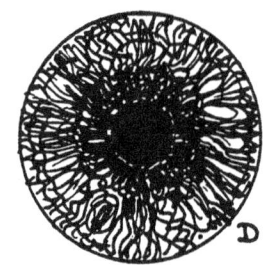

CAUSES:

REFINED CARBOHYDRATES.
MEATS FATS.
ALCOHOLS, SMOCKING.
DOMINATED PERSONS, WEAK CONSTITUTION.
IMBALANCED NUTRITION.
POOR ELIMINATION.
EMOTIONAL STRESS, FEAR, AWARNESS
ADRENAL IMBALANCE
BIRTH CONTROLL PILLS
LIVER, SPLEEN, KIDNEYS UNDER FUNCTION.
HYPOGLYCEMIA, DIABETES, LOW BLOOD PRESSURE.
CONSTIPATION

WHOLISTIC RELATION SHIPS.

NERVOUS & ENDOCRINE SYSTEMS
NERVOUS & DIGESTIVE SYSTEMS
NERVOUS & CIRCULATORY SYSTEMS.

TREATMENT

ADRENAL FORMULA (FD), PANCREAS FORMULA (FD)
ALKALINE FORMULA (FD)
BLOOD PURIFYING (DrC)
NERVE REJUVENATOR (FJD)
THYROID BALANCING FORMULA (FD)
BOWELS CLEANSING
GOOD FOOD COMBINING
WHOLE RICE, WHOLE WHEAT
FRESH RAW VEGETABLES
EXERCISE, REST, BREATHING EXERCISE.
RELAXATION EXERCISE.

O DESCENDING COLON (SEE CHART PAGE   )
O DESCENDING COLON DISEASES
        (SEE BOWELS CONDITIONS PAGE   )
        (SEE CONSTIPATION PAGE   )
O DIABETES
    IRIS SIGNS:
    A_ HESSIEN TYPE
        WEAK CONSTITUTION
        DILATED PUPIL
        DILATED ANW

    INDICATE: POOR BODY TONE.
        POOR MUSCLES.
        POOR ASSIMILATION.
        OBESTY OR OVER WEIGHT.
        INHERITED WEAKNESSES.
        CONSTIPATION.
        PRONE TO DIABETES.

    B _ LYMPHATIC TYPE
        DARK PANCREAS, SCURF RIM
        LIVER, KIDNEY, THYROID
         DISCOLORATIONS.
        WHITE BLADDER.
        DARK BOWELS RING
        ANW DISCOLORATION.
    INDICATE:
        TOXIC CIRCULATION.
        EXHAUSTED PANCREAS, LIVER, KIDNEY, THYROID.
        OVER ACTIVE BLADDER.
        CONSTIPATION.
        PRONE TO DIABETES.
    C _ LYMPHATIC TYPE
        DARK SCURF RIM THICK AT LOWER EXTREMETIES
        DARK KIDNEYS, BLADDER, PANCREAS, LIVER, EYE AND
         5 SENSES AREA, DARK THYROID.
    INDICATE:
        SEVERE DIABETIC CONDITION CAUSING VISION LOSS
            POOR CIRCULATION AT FEET (BLEEDING FEET)
            LIVER & KIDNEYS DAMAGE, ENDOCRINE IMBALANCE.
    D_ BROWN IRIS
        SAME CONDITIONS AND INDICATIONS OF IRIS C

    E _ DIABETES WHOLISTIC RELATIONSHIPS CHART
1_ ANIMATION LIFE, WILL POWER.
2_ PANCREAS
3_ LIVER RIGHT, SPLEEN LEFT
4_ LEGS, LOWER CIRCULATION
5_ ADRENALS
6_ KIDNEYS
7_ VAGINA, PENIS
8_ BLADDER
9_ EYE
10_ THYROID
11 _ LYMPH AND
   CAPILLARY CIRCULATION.
12_ DIGESTIVE TRACT.
13_ BLOOD SUPPLY

DIABETES

CAUSES:
REFINED CARBOHYDRATES
MEATS FATS
PANCREATIC EXHAUSTION
ENDOCRINE IMBALANCES
OVER WEIGHT
LIVER CONGESTION, LYMPH CONGESTION.
PROTEIN MALABSORBTION
ZINC, CHROMIUM DEFICIENCY
STRESS
MODERN CIVILIZATION
SEDENTARY LIFE STYLE
LACK OF PHYSICAL EXERCISE

WHOLISTIC RELATIONSHIPS
(SEE CHART PAGE D4)

TREATMENT:
WHOLE WHEAT RICH BRAN
WHOLE RICE
LENTILS
RAW FRESH VEGETABLES + GARLIC + ONIONS.
RICH NATURAL SOURCES OF ZINC, SELENIUM, CHROMIUM
VEGETABLE PROTEINS
PANCREAS FORMULA (FD)
ANTI-OBESE FORMULA (DrC)
BLOOD CIRCULATION FORMULAS A & B
PHYSICAL EXERCISE START GENTLY.

AVOID:
FRUITS FRESH & DRIED
FATS, MEATS, DAIRY.
OVER EATING, HEAVY MEALS.
FASTING
OVER BOILED VEGETABLES
CANNED FOOD
FRIED FOODS
WHITE SUGAR, MOLASSES, BROWN SUGAR, WHITE FLOUR.
POLISHED RICE
STRESS

O DIAPHRAGM (SEE CHART PAGE D11)

O DIARRHEA

IRIS SIGNS:
A - DIARRHEA CAUSED BY GASTRITIS
INDICATED BY WHITE FIBRES IN
STOMACH RING.
B - DIARRHEA CAUSED BY DILATED
ILEO CECAL VALVE
INDICATED BY WHITENESS IN THE
ICV. AREA.
WHITENESS IN THE PEYER'S PATCHES
AREA.

A   B
RIGHT

DIARRHEA.

CAUSES:
   OVER EATING
   GASTRITIS
   COLITIS
   INTESTINAL PARISITIS
   TOXICITY
   ENLARGED ILEO CECAL VALUE
   DRUGS, ANTI BIOTICS
   C VITAMIN EXCESS
   BRAN EXCESS
   CONTAMINATED WATER
   FOOD ALLERGY

WHOLISTIC RELATION SHIPS:
   DIGESTIVE & NERVOUS SYSTEMS
   DIGESTIVE & CIRCULATORY SYSTEMS
   DIGESTIVE & LYMPHIC SYSTEM.

TREATMENT:
   DEPENDS UPON THE CAUSES

O DIGESTIVE SYSTEM CHART (SEE PAGE D7)
O DIGESTIVE SYSTEM DISEASES
   SEE APPENDICITIS PAGE
   SEE BOWELS CONDITIONS PAGE
   SEE COLITIS PAGE
   SEE CONSTIPATION PAGE
   SEE DIARRHEA PAGE
   SEE DIVERTICULITIS PAGE D8
   SEE DUODENAL ULCER PAGE
   SEE GINGIVITIS PAGE
   SEE GALL BLADDER DISEASE PAGE
   SEE HEMORRHOIDS (PILES) PAGE
   SEE HEPATITIS PAGE
   SEE PYORRHIA PAGE
   SEE STOMACH ACIDITY PAGE
   SEE STOMACH ULCERS PAGE
   SEE STOMACH INFLAMMATIONS (GASTRITIS)

CHART TO IRIDOLOGY
DIGESTIVE SYSTEM

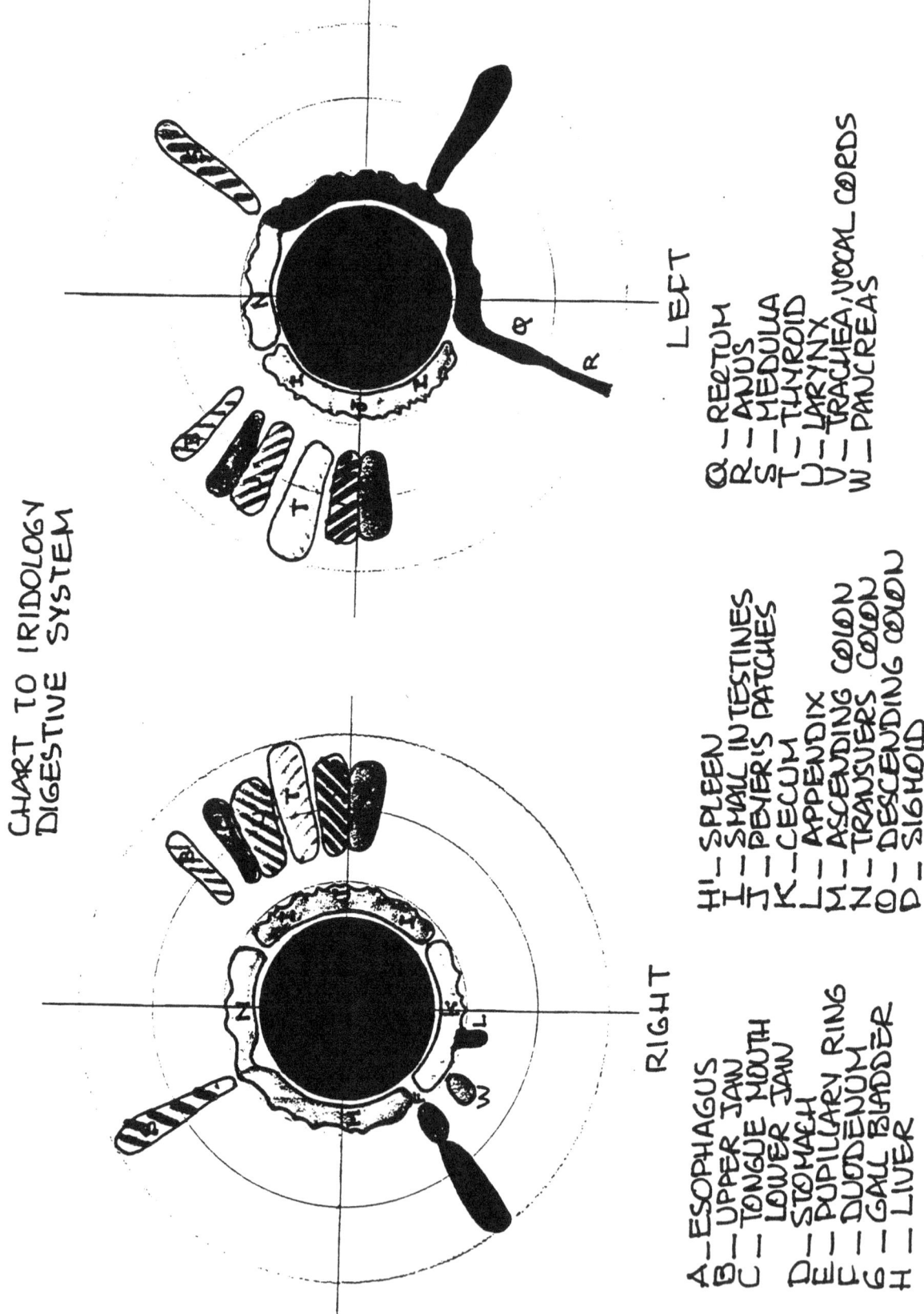

RIGHT

LEFT

A — ESOPHAGUS
B — UPPER JAW
C — TONGUE MOUTH
    LOWER JAW
D — STOMACH
E — PUPILLARY RING
F — DUODENUM
G — GALL BLADDER
H — LIVER

H — SPLEEN
I — SMALL INTESTINES
J — PEYER'S PATCHES
K — CECUM
L — APPENDIX
M — ASCENDING COLON
N — TRANSVERS COLON
O — DESCENDING COLON
P — SIGMOID

Q — RECTUM
R — ANUS
S — MEDULLA
T — THYROID
U — LARYNX
V — TRACHEA/VOCAL CORDS
W — PANCREAS

O DIVERTICULITIS (BOWELS POCKETS INFLAMMATION)

IRIS SIGNS:
DARK LACUNAE IN THE ANW
WHITE STREAKS IN THE LARGE
  INTESTINS AREA

INDICATIONS:
 CONSTIPATION
 CHRONIC BOWELS POCKETS
 INFLAMMATION OF THE LARGE INTESTINAL
  WALL

CAUSES:
 CHRONIC CONSTIPATION. (SEE CONSTIPATION CAUSES)
 OVER EATING.
 WEAKENED INTESTINAL WALL CAUSING THE FORMATION
  OF HERNIA.
 SLOW PERISTALSIC MUSCULAR ACTIVITY AND POOR
  BOWELS MOVEMENT, HELP THE SITE FOR PARASITIS
  AND BACTERIA TO ACCUMULATE INTO THE POCKETS
  CAUSING INFLAMMATION AND PAIN.

WHOLISTIC RELATION SHIPS
 DIGESTIVE & MUSCULAR SYSTEMS
 DIGESTIVE & CIRCULATORY SYSTEMS
 DIGESTIVE & URINARY SYSTEMS.

TREATMENT:
 CLEANSING PROGRAMES
 RECTAL BOLUS
 FASTING
 SEE ALSO CONSTIPATION TREATMENTS.

O DIZZINESS CENTRE (SEE CHART PAGE D11)
O DIZZINESS

IRIS SIGNS:
A - DIZZINESS CAUSED BY CEREBRAL
 WEAKNESS. INDICATED BY:
 DARK OR BROWN STREAKS
 RADIATING FROM THE CNS
 INTO DIZZINESS CENTRE
 AND EAR AREA.
B - DIZZINESS CAUSED BY
 CONSTIPATION AND IMPULSES
 FROM THE SPLENIC FLEXURE.
 INDICATED BY SQUARE SHAPED ANW.
C - DIZZINESS CAUSED BY EAR
 (INNER EAR) INFLAMMATION
 OR CONGESTED BLOOD
 SUPPLY. INDICATED BY WHITE
 FLARES OR LYMPHIC TOPHI
 IN THE EAR AREA. THE
 5 SENSE AREA MAY RECORD
 SOME WHITENESS AS WELL.
D - DIZZINESS CAUSED BY
 VENOUS CONGESTION AT THE
 BRAINS BLOOD SUPPLY. INDICATED BY BROWN CLOUDS
 IN THE VENOUS SUPPLY AREA. AND ARCUS SENILES.
 (SEE CHART PAGE A14)
 (SEE CHART PAGE C7).

47

DIZZINESS

E - DIZZINESS CASED BY
    ARTERIAL HARDNING
    ARTERIOSCLEROSIS IN THE
    HEAD AND EARS.
    INDICATED BY SODIUM RING
    PASSING THROUGH THE WHOLE
    HEAD AREA.

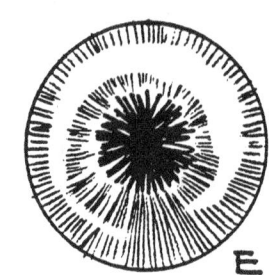

E

WHOLISTIC RELATION SHIPS
    NERVOUS & CIRCULATORY SYSTEMS
    NERVOUS & DIGESTIVE SYSTEMS
    NERVOUS & LYMPHIC SYSTEMS.
    NERVOUS & ENDOCRINE SYSTEMS.

TREATMENT:
    CASE A - CLEANS BOWELS
             NERVE TONICS.
    CASE B - TREAT CONSTIPATION
    CASE C - BLOOD PURIFICATION (FD)
             ANTI BIOTIC NATURAL (FD)
             ALKALINE FORMULA (FD)
    CASE D - BLOOD CIRCULATION (D-C) & (FD)
             ANAEMEA FORMULA (FD)
             BOUNCING.
    CASE E - TREAT CHOLESTEROL   DEPOSITS
             TREAT CIRCULATION
             ACID ALKALINE BALANCE.

O DRUGS DEPOSITS (PSORIC SPOTS)
IRIS SIGNS:
    COLOURED PIGMENTATIONS IN VARIOUS
        ORGANS AREAS.
INDICATIONS:
    ACCUMULATION OF DRUGS, CHEMICALS OR
    POLLUTION, IN THE ORGAN AREA.
    ACCUMULATION OF FAULTY METABOLIC
    BY-PRODUCT.

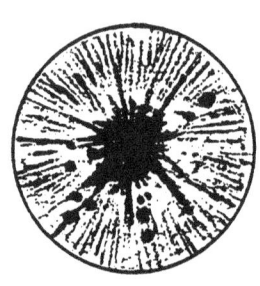

CAUSES:
    LONG ORTHODOX DRUGS THERAPY.
    POLLUTED OCCUPATION.
    INHERITED
    TOXIC BLOOD
    POOR ELIMINATION

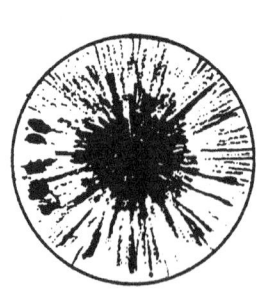

WHOLISTIC RELATION SHIPS:
    CIRCULATORY & ALL OTHER SYSTEMS.
TREATMENT:
    CLEANSING PROGRAMES.
    BLOOD PURIFICATIONS.
    FASTINGS.
    STIMULATE ALL ELIMINATIVE CHANNELS.

○ DUODENUM (SEE CHART PAGE D 11)
○ DUODENAL ULCER
  IRIS SIGNS:
    RAISED WHITE FIBERS IN THE DUODENUM AREA.
    SOME CASES RECORDS DARKNESS IN THE LIVER, PANCREAS
      AND GALL BLADDER AREAS.
  INDICATIONS:
    INFLAMMATION AT THE
      DUODENUM
    ULCERATION CONDITION IN THE
      DUODENUM.
  CAUSES:
    OVER SECRETIONS OF.
      PANCREATIC JUICES INTO THE
      DUODENUM.
    OVER SECRETIONS OF BILE.
    EXHAUSTED PANCREAS.
    HYPER ACID STOMACH.
    ACID ALKALINE IMBALANCE.
    OVER BOILED VEGETABLES.
    POLISHED RICE.
    FIBER DEFICIENCY.
    REFINED CARBOHYDRATES.
    SPASMS.
    EMOTIONAL STRESS
    POOR CHEWING.
    BAD FOOD COMBINING.

  WHOLISTIC RELATION SHIPS:
    DIGESTIVE & NERVOUS SYSTEMS
    DIGESTIVE & MUSCULAR SYSTEMS
    DIGESTIVE & ENDOCRINE SYSTEMS
  TREATMENTS:
    CABBAGE JUICE
    CARROT JUICE
    RAW POTATO JUICE
    LICORICE
    COMPHREY TEA.
  AVOID:
    COFFEE, TEA, ALCOHOLS.
    POLISHED RICE, SUGARS.
    MEATS, DAIRY.
    FRIED FOODS
    CITRIC FRUITS.
    PEPPERS
    VERY COLD DRINKS
    STRESS
    EMOTIONS
    SALTS
    SPICES

RIGHT IRIS

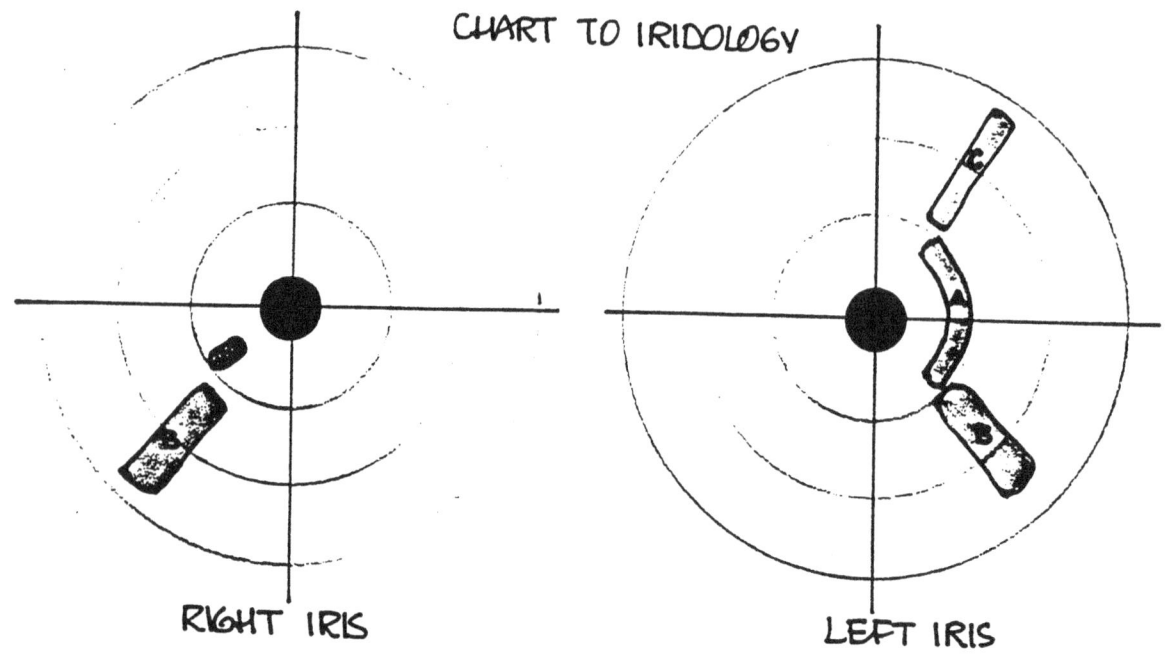

CHART TO IRIDOLOGY

RIGHT IRIS

LEFT IRIS

A - DESCENDING COLON.
B - DIAPHRAGM.
C - DIZZINESS CENTER.
D - DUODENUM.

BASED ON CHARTS TO IRIDOLOGY DEVELOPED BY
Dr. BERNARD JENSEN AND DOROTHY HALL.

O EAR (SEE CHART PAGE E1)
O EARACHE

A_ EARACHE CAUSED BY SINUS
   CONDITION, TONSILITIS
   AND FEVER.
   INDICATED BY:
    LYMPHIC ROSARY
    YELLOW_BROWN CLOUDS
    IN THE UPPER ANW AREA
    YELLOW BROWN TOPHI IN
    TONSILES AREA
    WHITE PEYER'S PATCHES
    MAY ALSO APPEAR.

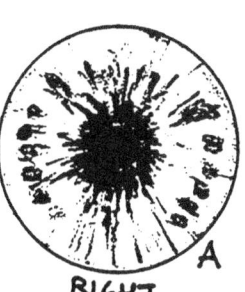
RIGHT   LEFT

B_ EARACHE CAUSED BY
   CONSTIPATION AND TOXIC
   SETTELMENTS IN THE
   HEPATIC OR SPLENATIC
   FLEXTURE CAUSING
   PAIN IMPULSES TO THE EAR.
   INDICATED BY:
   DARK BROWN BOWELS AREA
   RADII SOLERIS RADIATING INTO EAR AREAS.

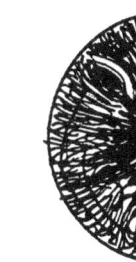
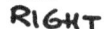
RIGHT   RIGHT

C_ EARACHE CAUSED BY HEADACHE
   INDICATED BY:
   EXHAUSTED LIVER DARK AREA
   NERVE RINGS IN HEAD AREAS
   CONGESTED BLOOD SUPPLY TO BRAIN

D_ EARACHE CAUSED BY CERVICAL UN ALIGNMENT
   INDICATED; BY WEAKNESS LESION IN THE NECK AREA
   WHITENESS IN EAR AREA, WEAK CONSTITUTION.

WHOLISTIC RELATION SHIPS:
   NERVOUS & LYMPHIC SYSTEMS
   NERVOUS & CIRCULATORY SYSTEMS
   NERVOUS & DIGESTIVE SYSTEMS
   NERVOUS & SKELETAL SYSTEMS

TREATMENT:
- IRIS A CONDITION:
   TREAT SINUSITIS AND ACIDIC CONDITIONS
   STIMULATE ELIMINATION
   ACID ALKALINE BALANCING
   (SEE ALSO ACIDITY TREATMENT.)
- IRIS B CONDITION:
   TREAT CONSTIPATION
- IRIS C CONDITION
   TREAT CONSTIPATION
   LIVER FLUSHING GALL BLADDER CLEANSING.
- IRIS D CONDITION
   CHIROPRACTICE, OSTEOPATHY, ALEXANDER TECHNIQUE.
   CALCIUM FORMULA (FD)
   EXERCISE
   SEDATIVES CAMMOMILE
   SWEET SLEEP FORMULA (FD)

O ECZEMA

IRIS SIGNS:

LYMPHIC ROSARY
DARK BOWELS
SCURF RIM
LYMPHIC TOPHI IN EXTREMITIES
 GROIN AND UNDER ARM.
IN SOME CONDITIONS: WEAKNESS
LESIONS IN LIVER & KIDNEYS AREAS

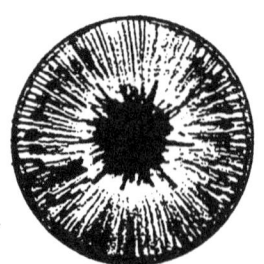

INDICATIONS:
LYMPHIC CONGESTION
CONSTIPATION
SLUGGISH SKIN, POOR CIRCULATION
UNDER FUNCTION LIVER TO PURIFY BLOOD
KIDNEYS WEAKNESS
POOR GENERAL ELIMINATION

CAUSES:
TOXIMIA   DUE TO POOR ELIMINATIVE CHANNELS
POOR SKIN RESPIRATION
ACID ACCUMULATION
POOR IMMUNE SYSTEM DUE TO LYMPH CONGESTION
OVER BURDENED LIVER AND KIDNEYS

WHOLISTIC RELATION SHIPS:
LYMPHIC & CIRCULATORY SYSTEMS
LYMPHIC & DIGESTIVE SYSTEMS
LYMPHIC & RESPIRATORY SYSTEMS

TREATMENT:
BOWELS CLEANSING
VEGETABLES JUICE FASTING.
BLOOD PURIFICATION (PD)
FUNEGREEK

O EGO PRESSURE AREA (SEE CHART PAGE E7)

O ELIMINATIVE CHANNELS

A _ BOWELS: ELIMINATE STOOL, TOXICS, METABOLIC
BY_PRODUCTS, FLUIDS, DIED CELLS

B _ LUNGS: ELIMINATE CARBON DI_OXIDE & WATER

C _ LYMPH: ELIMINATE TOXINS, DIED CELLS, WASTE
MATERIALS, METABOLIC BY_PRODUCTS, FATS

D _ KIDNEYS: ELIMINATE FLUIDS, TOXINS, METABOLIC
BY_PRODUCTS, WASTE MATERIALS

E _ SKIN: ELIMINATE TOXIC GASES, WATER, DIED
CELLS

O ELIMINATIVE CHANNELS CHART

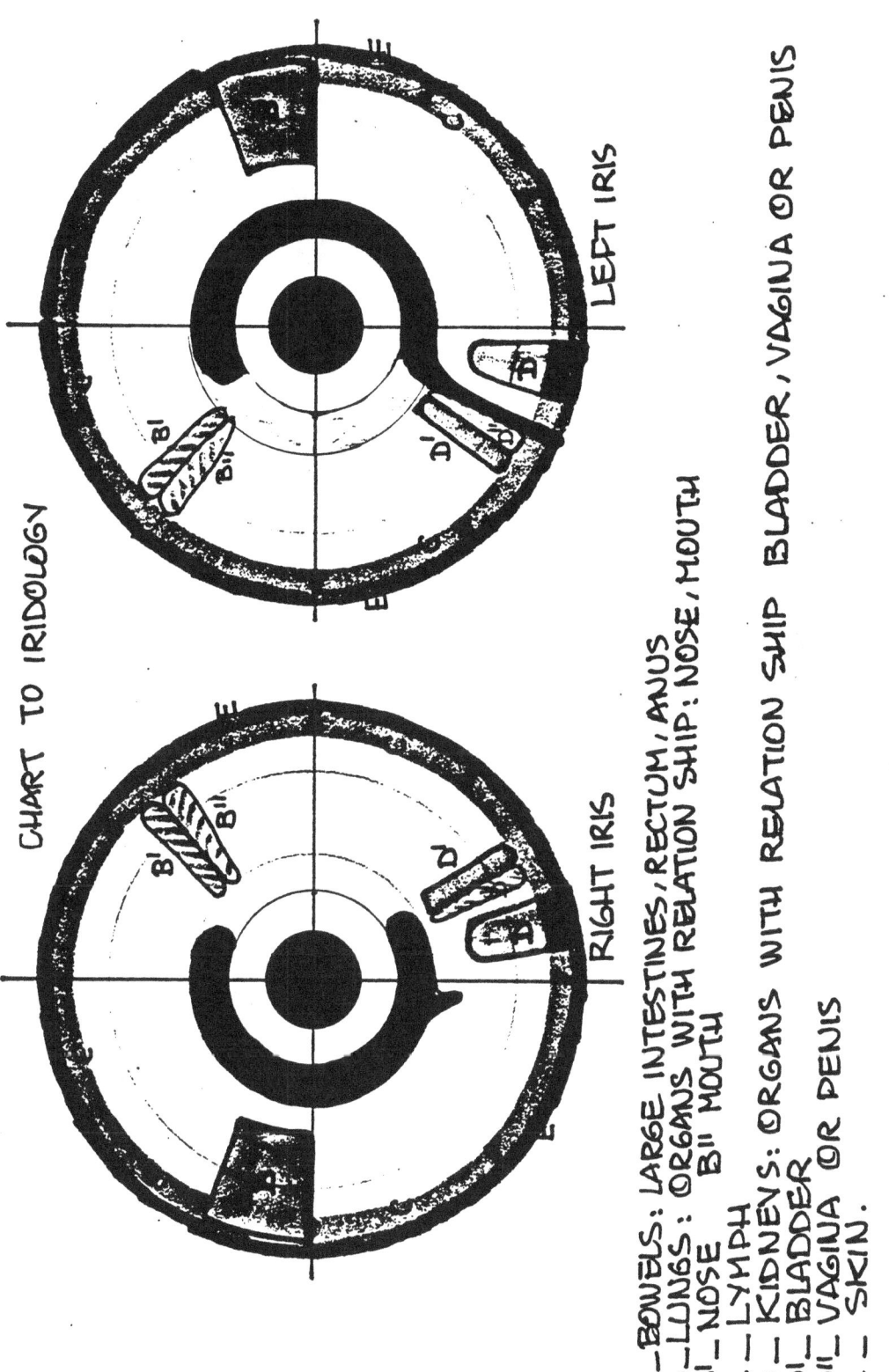

CHART TO IRIDOLOGY

RIGHT IRIS

LEFT IRIS

A.-BOWELS: LARGE INTESTINES, RECTUM, ANUS
B.-LUNGS: ORGANS WITH RELATION SHIP: NOSE, MOUTH
B'- NOSE   B'' MOUTH
C.- LYMPH
D.- KIDNEYS: ORGANS WITH RELATION SHIP BLADDER, VAGINA OR PENIS
D'- BLADDER
D''- VAGINA OR PENIS
E.- SKIN.

O ENDOCRINE SYSTEM CHART

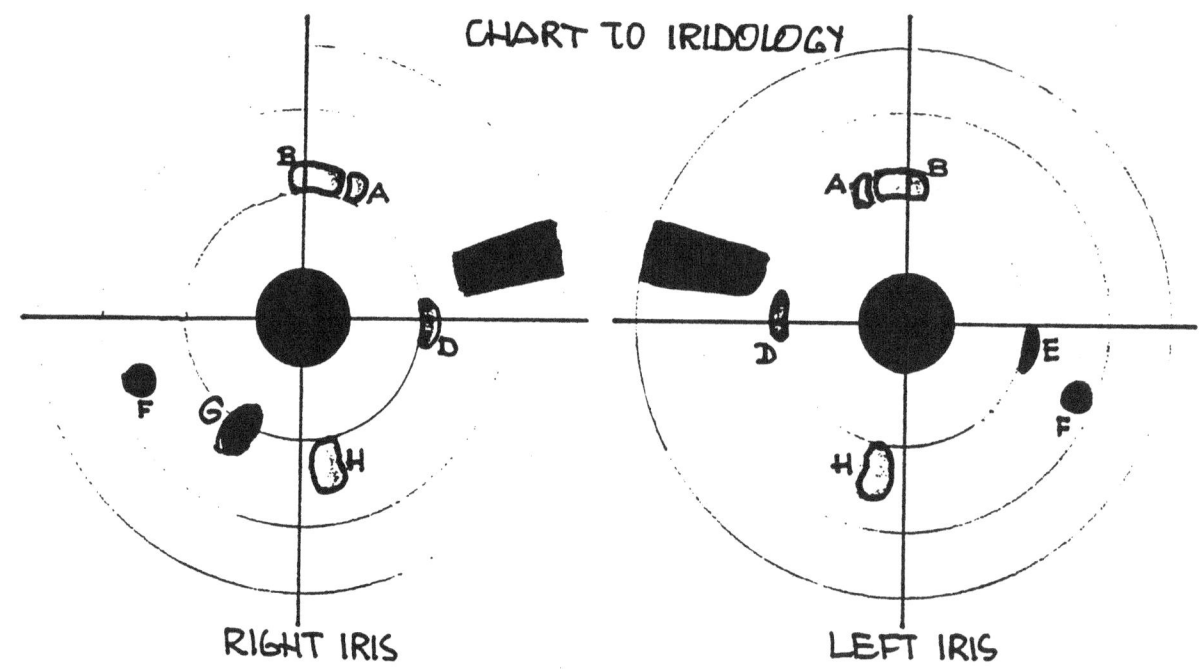

CHART TO IRIDOLOGY

RIGHT IRIS   LEFT IRIS

A — PINEAL GLAND
B — PITUITARY GLAND
C — THYROID GLAND
D — PARATHYROID GLAND
E — THYMUS GLAND
F — MAMMARY GLAND
G — PANCREAS
H — ADRENAL GLAND

O ENDOCRINE DISEASES

A — PINEAL GLAND
IRIS SIGNS:
VERY DARK TRANSVERSE COLON
RUST, YELLOW, BROWN IN UPPER CILIARY ZONE

INDICATIONS:
CONSTIPATION
TOXIC CONDITION OF TRANSVERSE COLON
SINUS CONGESTION
INHIBITED PINEAL FUNCTION

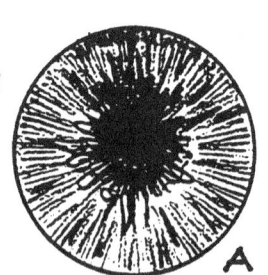

A

B — PITUITARY GLAND
IRIS SIGNS:
SAME IRIS CONDITIONS OF PINEAL GLAND
WEAKNESS SIGNS IN SKELETAL AREAS
NERVE RINGS IN SKELETAL AREAS

INDICATIONS:
CONSTIPATION, FAECES ACCUMULATION IN THE
TRANSVERSE COLON
SINUS CHRONIC CONDITION
WEAKNESS AND METABOLIC IRRITATION IN
THE SKELETAL SYSTEM
THYROID & ADRENAL ALSO INHIBITED IN FUNCTION
AS A RESULT OF PITUITARY IMBALANCE.

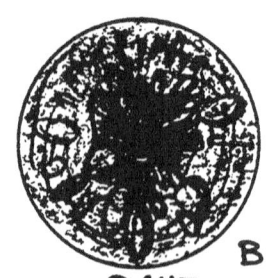

RIGHT

B

ENDOCRINE DISEASES
– THYROID GLAND
C – HYPER THYROIDISM
IRIS SIGNS:
WHITENESS IN THYROID AREA
SILK LINEN OR LINEN STRUCTURE
INDICATIONS:
GOOD CONSTITUTION, ENERGETIC
INSOMNIA, CONSTANT DOING
HYPER FUNCTION OF THYROID
FAST DIGESTION

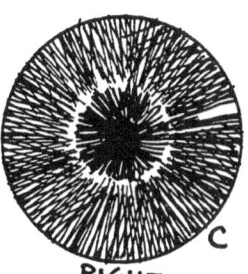

RIGHT   C

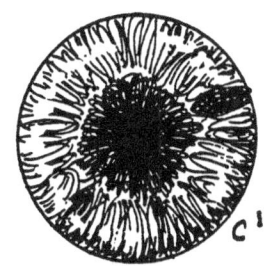

RIGHT   C¹

C¹ – HYPOTHYROIDISM
IRIS SIGNS:
WEAKNESS LESION IN THYROID AREA, LYMPH ROSARY
HESSIAN OR NET STRUCTURE
INDICATIONS:
LYMPH CONGESTION DUE TO CONSTIPATION AND
SLOW STAGNENT DIGESTION
HYPO FUNCTION OF THE THYROID

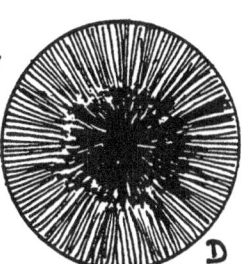

RIGHT   D

D – PARATHYROID
IRIS SIGNS:
BOWELS POCKETS IN SMALL INTESTINES
DARK ALIMANTARY CANAL
AND DISCOLORATIONS
INDICATIONS:
CONSTIPATION
TOXIC CIRCULATION
HYPOFUNCTION OF THE PARATHYROID GLAND

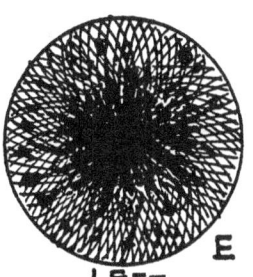

LEFT   E

E – THYMUS GLAND
IRIS SIGNS:
YELLOW–BROWN LYMPHIC TOPH IN THYMUS AREA
LYMPHIC ROSARY
HESSIEN STRUCTURE.
INDICATIONS:
POOR IMMUNITY, LYMPHIC CONGESTION
INHIBITED THYMUS FUNCTION.

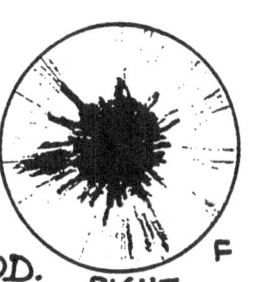

RIGHT   F

F – MAMMARY GLANDS
IRIS SIGNS:
YELLOW–BROWN CLOUDS IN MAM. GLANDS INDICATE
TOXINS ACCUMULATIONS, WHITENESS INDICATE A
GOOD SIGN OF HEALTHY BREAST FEEDING PERIOD.

G – PANCREAS
IRIS SIGNS: (SEE ALSO DIABETES)
WHITE SIGNS IN THE PANCREAS AREA INDICATE
AN ACUTE HYPOGLYCIMIC CONDITION
DARK DIAMOND SHAPED INDICATE INHIBITED
FUNCTION, EXHAUSTION AND EVENTUALLY
HIGH BLOOD SUGAR (DIABETES).

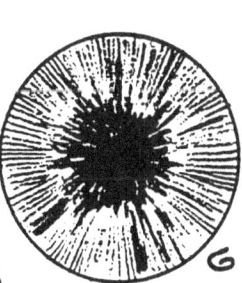

G

H – ADRENAL GLAND
IRIS SIGNS:
DARK BOWELS AREA, POCKETS CECUM & OR SIGMOID
DARK LINES IN ADRENAL AREA
DILATED PUPIL
INDICATIONS:
CONSTIPATION, ADRENAL EXHAUSTION
DEPRESSION, FEAR

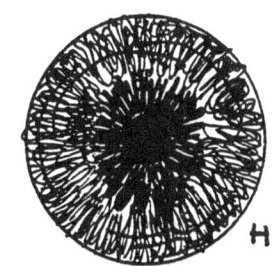

H

ENDOCRINE DISEASES

CAUSES:

INHERITED WEAKNESS LESIONS
POOR CIRCULATION
POOR OXYGENATION
IMPROPER DIET
MEAT, DAIRY, FATS EXCESS
CONSTIPATION
TOXICITY
RAW FRESH VEGETABLES DEFICIENCY
SEDENTARY OCCUPATION
LACK OF PHYSICAL ACTIVITY
LACK OF BODY TONE
STRESS
NERVOUSNESS

WHOLLISTIC RELATIONSHIPS:

ENDOCRINE & CIRCULATORY SYSTEMS
ENDOCRINE & DIGESTIVE SYSTEMS
ENDOCRINE & NERVOUS SYSTEMS
ENDOCRINE & SKELETAL SYSTEMS
ENDOCRINE & URINARY SYSTEMS

TREATMENTS:

BOWELS CLEANSING, STIMULATE ELIMINATION.
EXERCISE
BLOOD PURIFICATION   (Dr.C)
BLOOD CIRCULATION (FD & Dr.C)
THYROID FORMULA (FD)
ADRENAL FORMULA (FD)
ALKALINE FORMULA (FD)
CALCIUM FORMULA (FD)
PANCREAS FORMULA (FD)

O ESOPHAGUS (SEE CHART PAGE E7)

O EQUILIBRIUM CENTER (SEE CHART PAGE E7)

O EYE (SEE CHART PAGE E7)

O EYE DISEASES

CHART TO IRIDOLOGY

RIGHT

LEFT

A — EAR
B — EGO PRESSURE
C — ESOPHAGUS
D — EQUILIBRIUM
E — EYE

O FACE AREA OF THE IRIS (SEE CHART PAGE F4)
O FATIGUE AREA (SEE CHART PAGE F4)
O FATIGUE
  A_IRIS SIGNS:
    ARCUS SENILES
    LOWER EXTREMITIES ANEMEA
  INDICATION:
    POOR BLOOD SUPPLY TO BRAIN
    AND ETREMITIES AREAS
    FATIGUE CAUSED BY ANEMEA
    CONDITIONS.
  B_IRIS SIGNS:
    RADII SOLERIS RADIATING FROM
    CNS INTO WILL POWER (FATIGUE)
    AREA, FEET, MEDULLA, LUNGS.
  INDICATIONS:
    FATIGUE AND WEAK WILL POWER
    CAUSED BY CONSTIPATION AND
    OXYGENATION

A   B

CAUSES:
    ANEMIA
    HYPOGLYCEMIA
    TOXICITY
    ENDOCRINE IMBALANCES
    POOR ELIMINATION
    IMPROPER DIET
    EXCESS OR INADEQUATE NUTRIENTS
    EXCESS SEX
    INSOMNIA
    STRESS
    DEGENARATIVE DISEASES
    LACK OF PHYSICAL ACTIVITY
    POOR BREATHING, MEDULLA WEAKNESS
    CONSTIPATION
    SCURVY
    E VITAMIN DEFICIENCY, B VIT. FAMILY DEFICIENCY.
    EXCESS BOILED OILS, DRIED FOODS.

WHOLISTIC RELATION SHIPS:
    ALL SYSTEMS INVOLVED
TREATMENTS:
    TREAT ANEMEA, TREAT BLOOD CIRCULATION.
    TREAT CONSTIPATION
    MULTI MINERALS & VITAMINS NATURAL (FD)
    C VITAMIN, E VITAMIN, B FAMILY VITAMINS
    ZINC, CHROMIUM, SELENIUM
    RETAIN OXYGEN (E VIT.)
    SWEET SLEEP FORMULA (FD)
    EXERCISE, REST, BREATHING EXERCISE.
    AVOID: OILS & FATS,
        MEATS, DAIRY, BREAD, SUGAR.
        HEAVY MEALS.
        OVER WORK.
        OVER SLEEP.
        STRESS.

O FEAR

IRIS SIGNS:
DILATED PUPIL
DILATED ANW
ADRENAL DISCOLORATION
DEEP NERVE RINGS.

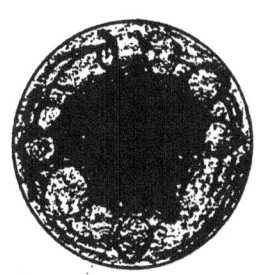

INDICATIONS:
SYMPATHETIC DOMINANCE
SWINGING ADRENALIN SECRETIONS
ADRENAL EXHAUSTION.
NERVOUS IRRITATION
SLOW DIGESTION

CAUSES:
HYPOGLYCEMIA.
STARCHY FOODS EXCESS.
FAT EXCESS.
PROTEIN DEFICIENCY.
RAW FRESH VEGETABLES DEFICIENCY.
CONSTIPATION.
POLLUTION.
INHERITED ADRENAL WEAKNESS.
MINERALS IMBALACES.
MAGNESIUM DEFICIENCY.
C VITAMIN & B FAMILY DEFICIENCY.
STRESS, INSOMNIA.

WHOLISTIC RELATION SHIPS:
NERVOUS & DIGESTIVE SYSTEMS
NERVOUS & CIRCULATORY SYSTEMS
NERVOUS & MUSCULAR SYSTEMS
NERVOUS & ENDOCRINE SYSTEMS

TREATMENTS:
STIMULATE ELIMINATIONS
NERVE TONIC (Dr C)
ADRENAL FORMULA (FD)
RELAXATIONS EXERCISES
MEDITATION
PHYSICAL EXERCISE
MULTI MINERALS / VITAMINS NATURALLY (FD)
FRESH VEGETABLES.
VEGETABLE PROTEINS

O FEET (SEE CHART PAGE F4)

O FEVER

IRIS SIGNS:
RAISED WHITE FIBERS IN ORGANS
AREA.
DARK BOWELS AREA.
RAISED WHITE FIBRES IN PEYER'S
PATCHES AREA.
IN SOME CASES SCURF RIM EXISTS.
RISA REVEALS ACUTE THROAT INFECTION
WHITE RADIALS IN TONSILS AREA AND WHITE
PEYER'S PATCHES. LYMPH ROSARY.

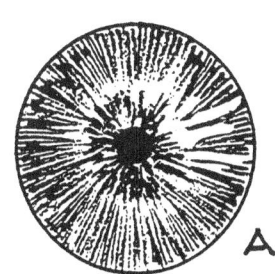

A

FEVER

CAUSES:
TOXICS ACCUMULATION.
HIGH ACIDIC LEVEL.
LYMPHIC CONGESTION.
INFLAMMATIONS.
ACUTE STAGES OF DISEASE
POOR FLUIDS ABSORBTION
CONSTIPATION, POOR ELIMINATION
VERY RICH NOURISHING FOODS
LACK OF FRESH VEGETABLES

WHOLISTIC RELATION SHIPS:
LYMPHATIC CIRCULATORY & ALL SYSTEMS.
TREATMENTS:
WATER FAST.
VEGETABLES BROTH FAST.
POTOTO PEELS WITH GARLIC BROTH FAST.
STIMULATE ELIMINATIVE CHANNELS
BOWELS CLEANSING
ANTIBIOTIC NATURALLY (FD)

O FIBER PATTERN OF IRIS
A_ SILK PATTERN / DENSITY 1
GOOD CONSTITUTION, HEALTHY BORN, RECOVER QUICKLY,
UN_DESIGNED TO LIVE WITH PLASTIC SOCIETIES,
STRONG, EARTH LOVERS, DIRECT LOOK ON LIFE,
SKILLED BUILDERS, THEY REPRESENT THE ANT'S
SOCIETY IN THE HUMAN KINGDOM.

B_ SILK_LINEN / DENSITY 2
GOOD CONSTITUTION, PRACTICAL ECONOMIC
PEOPLE, THEY CONCENTRATE WELL ON DOING
THEIR JOB. THEY ARE STRONG AND HEALTHY
HOWEVER THEY ARE PRONE TO ACID ACCUMULATION
ARTHRITIS AND KIDNEY STONES.

C_ THE LINEN IRIS / DENSITY 3
SOCIAL, DIPLOMATIC AND CO-OPERATIVE
AVERAGE STRENGTH, THEY LIKE REST AFTER
WORK. ABLE TO FEEL WITH OTHERS.
THEY ARE AWARE OF THEIR BODIES TOLERANCE.
THEY ACCEPT HELP WHEN OFFERED.
WEAKER IN CONSTITUTION AND PHYSICAL
STRUCTURE THAN THE FIRST TWO TYPES.
LESS RESISTANCE TO OVERCOME DISEASE

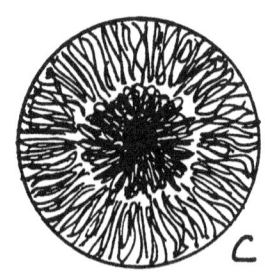

D_ THE HESSIAN TYPE IRIS / DENSITY 4
TENDENCY TO BUILD AND INVENT EQUIPMENT
THEY ASK FOR HELP AND ACCEPT IT WHEN
OFFERED.
   WEAKER CONSTITUTION AND STRENGTH
THAN THE LINEN IRIS, WEAKER RESISTANCE
TO DISEASE. UN PRONE TO PHYSICAL ACTIVITY
THEY FEEL DOMINATED.

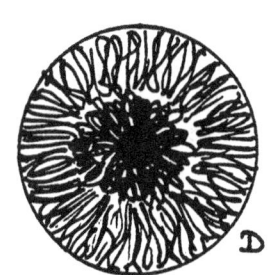

E_ THE NET IRIS / DENSITY 5
THEY INTELLIGENTLY COPE WITH THE AVAILABLE
LIVING QUALITIES.
CONTROLLED ENDURANCE NOT ENTIRELY
PHYSICAL. THEY ADJUST THEIR STRENGTH
ACCORDING TO THE APPROPRIATE DEMAND
      MYSTERIOUS BEHAVIOR WHEN UNDER
STRESS WHICH PROBABLY TOUCH THEIR
DIGNITY.

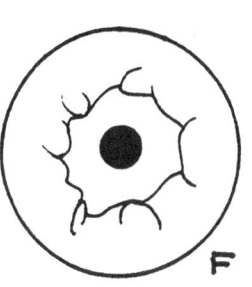

F_ BROWN IRIS / NO FIBERS   VISIBLE.
CONSTITUTION OF THE BROWN IRIS CAN BE
DETECTED THROUGH THE ANW CONDITION.
   DIGESTION DEFICIENCY, PRONE TO DISEASES
OF THE DIGESTIVE SYSTEM AND KIDNEYS
   THEIR ENERGY IS NOT FROM THE
MUSCULAR SYSTEM, IT IS ALMOST NERVOUS
ENERGY.

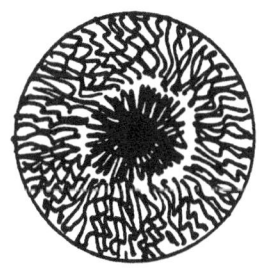

O FLATULANCE (SEE CONSTIPATION PAGE C10)
O FRUSTRATION
   IRIS SIGNS:
   ZIG ZAG FIBERS INDICATE FRUSTRATION
   OF AVAILABLE ENERGY FLOW.
   USUALLY ZIG ZAG FIBERS NEVER COVER THE
   WHOLE IRIS AREA. HOWEVER IT REVEALS THE
   FRUSTRATION CONDITION OF THE ORGAN AREA.

   F CHART TO IRIDOLOGY.

   A_FATIGUE AREA (WILL)
   B_FACE AREA
   C_FEET.

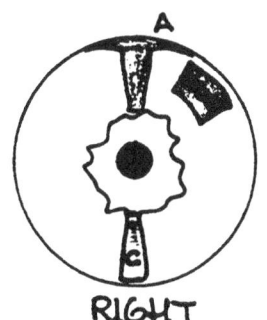
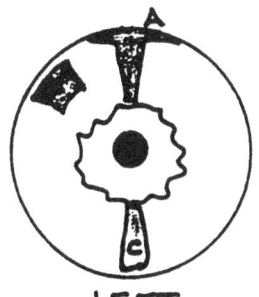

RIGHT   LEFT

O GALL BLADDER (SEE CHART PAGE 64)
O GALL BLADDER CONDITIONS

A_ IRIS SIGNS:
 WHITE OR YELLOW WHITE
 CLOUD IN THE GALL BLADDER
 AREA
 INDICATE:
 CHOLECYSTITIS, INFLAMMATION
 OF THE GALL BLADDER AND
 THE BILE DUCT

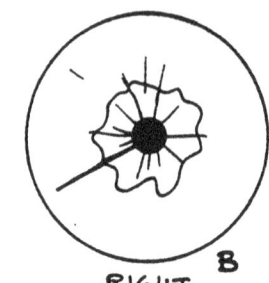
RIGHT   A

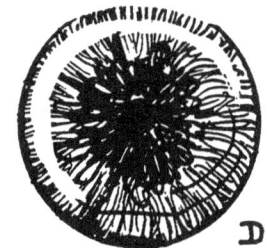
RIGHT   B

B_ STRONG RADIAL RADIATING
 FROM THE PUPIL PASSING INTO
 GALL BLADDER & LIVER
 INDICATE: A CHRONIC GALL
 BLADDER CONDITION AFFECTING
 THE CENTRAL NERVOUS SYSTEM

C_ VERY DARK GALL BLADDER
 AREA NERVE RINGS IN LIVER
 AREA, SCURF RIM, DARK BOWEL
 INDICATION:
 GALL BLADDER DEGENERATIVE
 CONDITION AND GALL STONES
 SUSPECTION. IRRITATED LIVER AND DIMINISHED FUNCTION
 CAUSING BLOOD TOXICITY. CONSTIPATION.

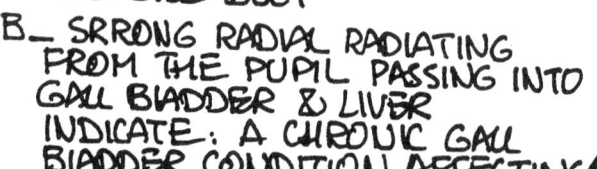
RIGHT   C

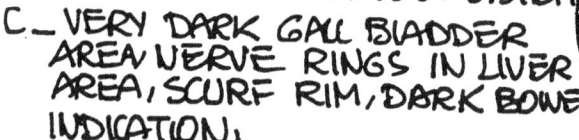
LEFT   D

D_ SODIUM RING, DARK BOWELS, SCURF RIM, DARK SPOTS
 IN THE ANUS AREA.
 INDICATE:
 CHOLESTEROLE ACCUMULATION, CHRONIC CONSTIPATION
 HEMORRHOIDS CAUSED AFTER THE REMOVAL OF THE
 GALL BLADDER. BRAIN ANEMIA MAY EXIST.

CAUSES:
 CONSTIPATION AND ALL THE CAUSES OF CONSTIPATION.
 HYDROGENATED FATS EXCESS.
 SATURATED FATS EXCESS.
 LACK OF VEGETABLES.
 LACK OF OLIVE OIL.
 OBESITY.
 POOR LYMPH & CIRCULATION.
 TOXIC LADENED BLOOD CAUSES OVER WORK TO LIVER
  EVENTUALLY DETERIORATE THE GALL BLADDER.

HOLISTIC RELATION SHIPS:
 DIGESTIVE & CIRCULATORY SYSTEMS
 DIGESTIVE & LYMPHIC SYSTEMS
 DIGESTIVE & NERVOUS SYSTEMS

TREATMENT:
 LIVER FLUSH, GALL BLADDER CLEANSING.
 BOWELS CLEANSING, STIMULATE ELIMINATIONS.
 GALL BLADDER CLEANSE FORMULA (FRANK ROBERTS)
 STRICT VEGAN DIET IS RECOMMANDED.
 CASTOR OIL PACKS.

O GANGRENE

IRIS SIGNS:
GANGRENE CONDITION IS UN DETECTED DIRECTLY
BY IRIS READING.

1. A THICK DARK SCURF RIM
   INDICATE A CONDITION PRONE
   TO GANGRENE

2. A DIABETIC CONDITION LEAD TO
   GANGRENE CONDITIOUS.

3. ANEMIA OF THE EXTREMETIES LEAD TO
   GANGRENE CONDITION.

4. SCURVY & E VITAMIN DEFICIENCY CAUSE GANGRENE.

5. SCURVY AND PYORRHEA CAUSE GANGRENE.

O GASTRITIS

IRIS SIGNS:
WHITE SIGNS IN THE STOMACH AREA.
INDICATE: INFLAMMATION OF THE MUCUS
MEMBRANE OF THE STOMACH.

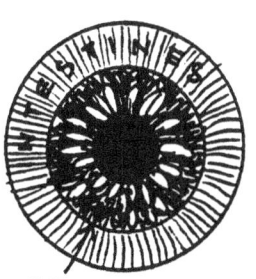

STOMACH

CAUSES:
EXCESS HCL.
EXCESS EMOTIONAL STRESS.
EXCESS ACID FORMING FOOD.
A VITAMIN DEFICIENCY.
POOR CHEWING
BAD FOOD COMBINING.
ADDITIVES, COLORINGS EXCESS
FRIED FOODS
POLISHED RICE.
FIBER DEFICENCY.

TREATMENT:
MONO DIET JUICE FASTS
ALKALINE FORMULA (FD)
RAW CABBAGE, RAW CARROTS.

O GASTRIC ULCER

IRIS SIGNS:
BLACK POINTS OR LINES IN THE STOMACH AREA
INDICATION:
GASTRIC ULCER.

CAUSES:
EXCESS ACID
UN TREATED ACUTE STOMACH ACIDITY
CONSTIPATION
LOW BLOOD SUGAR
PARASITIS
EXCESS CITRUS FRUITS JUICES
EXCESS SPICES
STRESS
POOR CHEWING, POOR DIGESTION
OVER BOILED VEGETABLES
SUGAR & POLISHED RICE.

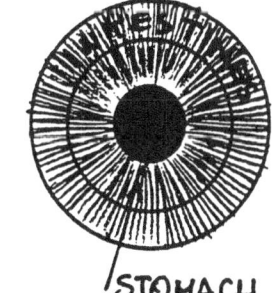

STOMACH

GASTRIC ULCER.

WHOLISTIC RELATION SHIPS:
DIGESTIVE & NERVOUS SYSTEMS
DIGESTIVE & MUSCULAR SYSTEMS
DIGESTIVE & ENDOCRINE SYSTEMS
DIGESTIVE & CIRCULATORY SYSTEMS

TREATMENT:
CABBAGE & CARROT JUICE FAST.
RAW POTATO JUICE
BOWELS CLEANSING
ANEMIA FORMULA (FD) AFTER HEALING.
AVOID: (SEE DUODENAL ULCER PAGE D10)

O GENITO URINARY AREA (SEE CHART PAGE G4)

O GLAOCOMA (SEE EYE DISEASES)

O GOITER (SEE THYROID GLAND PAGE T3)

O GOUT

IRIS SIGNS:
WHITE COLOURS IN THE CIRCULATORY
ZONE
INDICATION:
URIC ACID DIATHESIS TYPE.
ACCUMULATION OF URIC ACID
CRYSTALES.
PRONE TO ARTHRITIS AND
KIDNEY STONES.

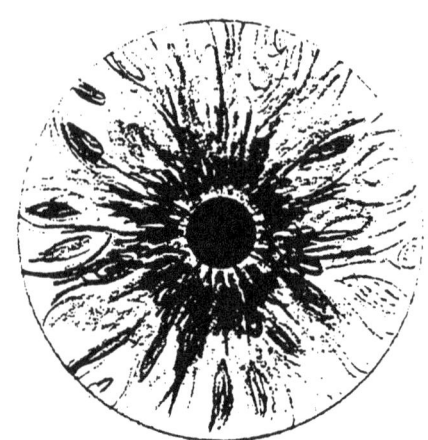

CAUSES:
MEATS CONSUMPTION EXCESS
REFINED STARCHES EXCESS
COFFEE, CHOCOLETS EXCESS
ENZYMES DEFICIENCIES.
ACID ALKALINE IMBALANCES
POOR ELIMINATIONS OF KIDNEYS, SKIN, LUNGS, LYMPH.
CONSTIPATION
SEDATIVE LIFE STYLE
ENDOCRINE IMBALANCES
POOR CIRCULATION
FRESH VEGETABLES DEFICIENCY
FLUIDS DEFICIENCY

WHOLISTIC RELATION SHIPS
CIRCULATORY & MUSCULAR SYSTEMS
CIRCULATORY & SKELETAL SYSTEMS
CIRCULATORY & DIGESTIVE SYSTEMS
CIRCULATORY & ENDOCRINE SYSTEMS
CIRCULATORY & LYMPHIC SYSTEMS.

GOUT

TREATMENT:
BOWELS CLEANSING
GALL BLADDER CLEANSING
KIDNEYS CLEANSING
MONO DIET JUICE FAST
VEGETABLE BROTH FAST
CELERY & PARSLEY JUICE
ALKALINE FORMULA (FD)
ADRENAL FORMULA (FD)
BLOOD CIRCULATION (FD)
THYROID FORMULA (FD)
AFTER RECOVERY:
FOLLOW A PERMANENT VEGAN DIET
EXERCISE
SKIN BRUSHING
SUN BATHING
CASTOR OIL PACKS.

O GROIN (SEE CHART PAGE 64)

G: CHART TO IRIDOLOGY

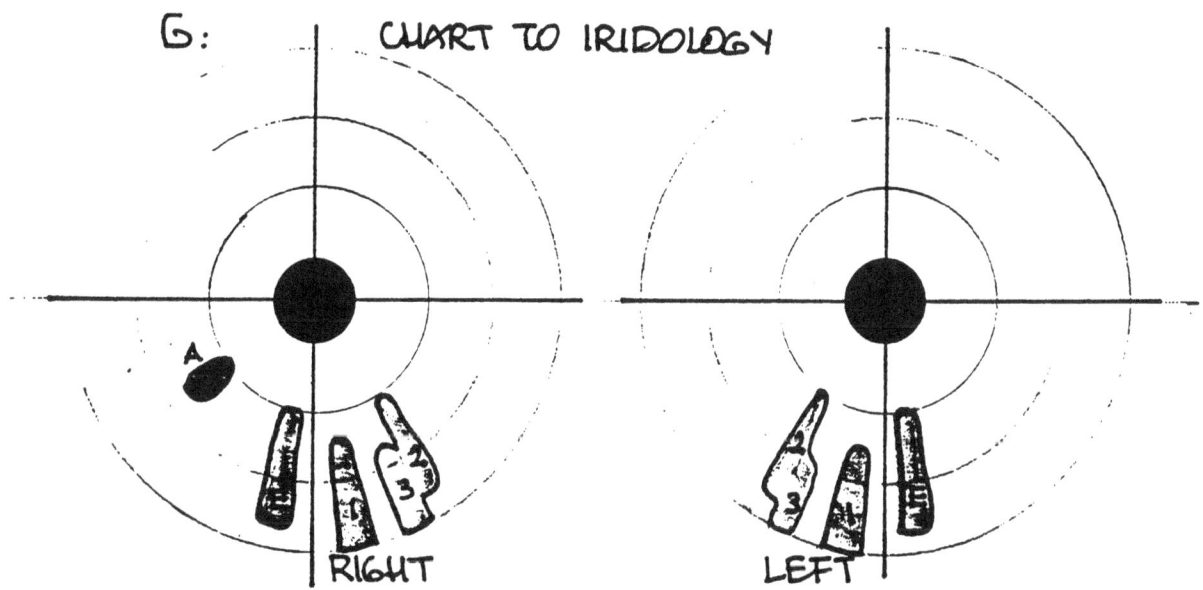

RIGHT   LEFT

A_GALL BLADDER
B_GASTRO_INTESTINAL AREA. SEE DIGESTIVE SYSTEM
C_GENITO URINARY AREA
    1.KIDNEY . 2_BLADDER. 3_PENIS OR VAGINA.
D_GLANDULAR SYSTEM. SEE ENDOCRINE SYSTEM
    AND REPRODUCTIVE SYSTEM
E_GROIN.

O HAND (SEE CHART PAGE H9)
O HARDENING OF THE ARTERIES
(SEE ARTERIOSCLEROSIS)

O HEAD ACHE
HEAD ACHE AND MIGRANE HAVE NO SPECIAL SIGN IN THE IRIS.
CONTRIBUTING FACTORS SHOULD BE DETECTED.

A _ HEAD ACHE CAUSED BY CONSTIPATION
AND FAECES SETTELMENTS IN
THE TRANSVERSE COLON.
INDICATED: BY HETEROCHROMIA IN UPPER
ANW.
NERVE RINGS IN BRAIN AREA
SINUSITIS CONDITION MAY EXIST.

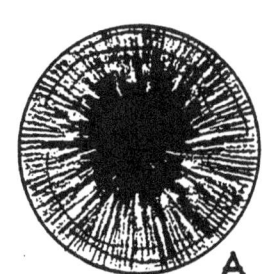
A

B _ HEAD ACHE CAUSED BY LIVER CONGESTION
INDICATED BY WEAKNESS LESIONS IN LIVER
AND GALL BLADDER AREAS.
NERVE RINGS.

C _ HEAD ACHE CAUSED BY CERVICAL
LESIONS.
INDICATED BY: BROWNISH RADIAL IN THE
NECK AREA.
NERVE RINGS FROM NECK TO HEAD AREAS.
BACK WEAKNESS MAY EXIST.

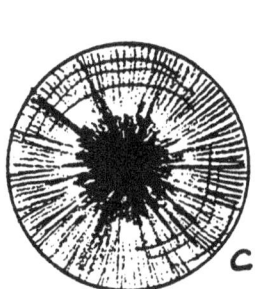
B

OTHER CAUSES:
EARS TROUBLES
VISION TROUBLES
INSOMNIA
VERY HOT AND/OR VERY COLD WEATHER
ULCERS
INTESTINAL PARASITIS
SINUSITIS
CONSTIPATION
POOR BREATHING/MEDULLA WEAKNESS
DRUGS
EMOTIONAL STRESS
ANXIETY, FEAR.
FRUSTRATIONS
AND MANY OTHERS.

WHOLISTIC RELATIONSHIPS.
NERVOUS SYSTEM AND ALL SYSTEMS.

TREATMENT:
DEPENDS UPON CAUSES, CONSTITUTIONAL TYPE
AND CONTRIBUTING FACTORS.

C

O HEAD AREA (SEE CHART PAGE 49)

O HEALING SIGNS

A _ IRIS SIGNS:
   BRIGHTNESS OF
   COLOURS.
   LIGHT.
   DARKNESS _
   DISAPPEARANCE.

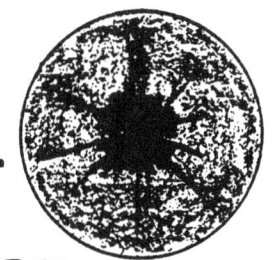

A

BEFORE TREATMENT   AFTER TREATMENT.

B _ IRIS SIGNS:
   BLUE IRIS
   HEALING OF BRONCHIAL TROUBLE
   INDICATED BY WHITE LINES
   FILLING THE DARK LESION IN
   LUNGS & BRONCHIAL AREA

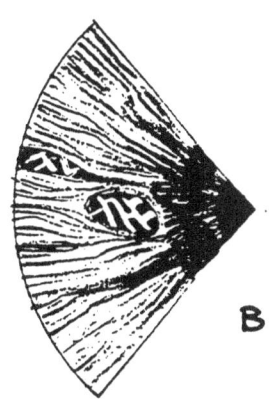

B

C _ IRIS SIGNS:
   WHITENESS & BRIGHTNESS OF LYMPHIC ROSARY.
   TRANSFORMATION FROM DARK BROWN TO LIGHT
   ORANGE AFTER CLEANSING AND ELIMINATIVE
   PROGRAME.

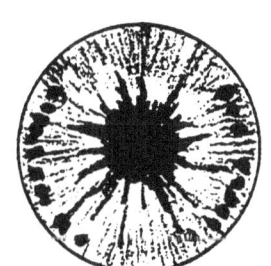

C

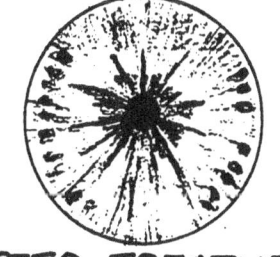

BEFORE TREATMENT   AFTER TREATMENT

O HEART AREA (SEE CHART PAGE H9)
O HEART CONDITIONS

A_ ENDOCARDITIS: INFLAMMATION OF THE ENDOCARDIUM
    INDICATED BY:
    SMALL WHITE FLAKES IN THE HEART AREA.
    SHORT WHITE LINES CLOSE TO THE ANW.

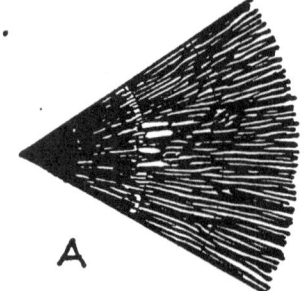

A

B_ MYOCARDITIS: INFLAMMATION
        OF THE HEART MUSCLES.
    INDICATED BY:
    SMALL WHITE FLAKES IN THE MUSCLE
    ZONE IN THE MIDDLE OF THE HEART
    OR FURTHER OUTWARDS TOWARDS THE
    SKELETAL ZONE.

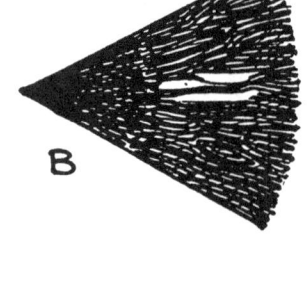

B

C_ PERICARDITIS: INFLAMMATION OF THE
        PERICARDIUM.
    INDICATED BY:
    WHITE CLOUDS IN THE LOWER MARGIN
    OF THE HEART.
    WHITE ADHESION SIGNS, TRANSVERSALS

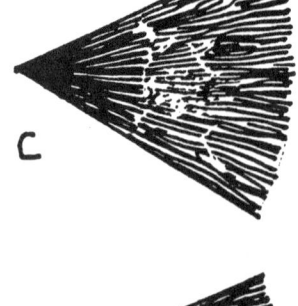

C

D_ CARDIAC NEUROSES: NERVOUS
        DISTURBANCES OF THE HEART.
    INDICATED BY:
    VERY FINE WHITE LINE WHICH RUNS OUT
    OVER THE HEART AREA FROM THE
    IRIS WREATH, ROUGHLY HORIZONTALLY

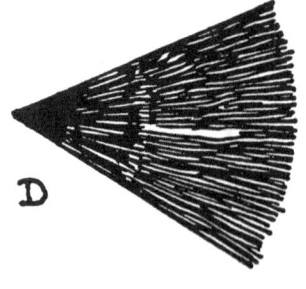

D

E_ CARDIAC NEUROSES
    WITH STRONGER NERVOUS DISTURBANCE
    INDICATED BY:
    ZIG ZAG FORM WHITE LINE REFLEXIVE FIBRE
    NERVE RINGS
    THIS CONDITION CONTRIBUTES TO
    THE RISK CARDIAC SPASM AND THE
    APPEARANCE OF PRAECORDIAL
    ANGINAL ATTACKS.

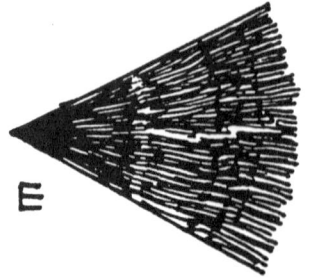

E

HEART CONDITIONS

F — CARDIAC MYASTHENIA: HEART MUSCLE WEAKNESS

INDICATED BY:
DARK HEART AREA, AS DARK WISPS CLOUDS OR CLOSED OR OPEN LESIONS

THE WIDER THE SEPARATION OF THE FIBRES IN THE HEART AREA, THE GREATER THE TENDENCY TO CARDIAC DILATION.

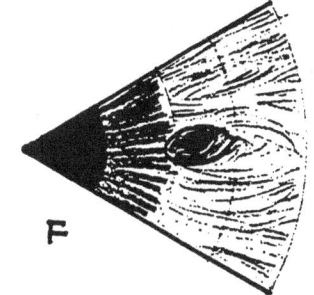

F

G — CARDIAC VALVE LESIONS:

INDICATED BY:
SMALL BLACK POINTS IN THE HEART AREA IN THE VICINITY OF THE ANW LYING IN THE UPPER PART OF THE AREA.
THERE MAY BE ONE TO THREE BLACK POINTS. THE APPEARANCE OF A FORTH POINTS IS A PRESAGE OF DEATH.

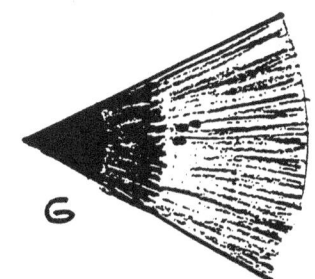

G

H — CORONARY SCLEROSIS:

INDICATED BY:
THICK WHITE MARGIN, COINJOINED WITH THE LOWER ARC OF A CARDIAC WEAKNESS SIGN, AND EXTENDED WITH IT TO THE MUSCLE ZONE.

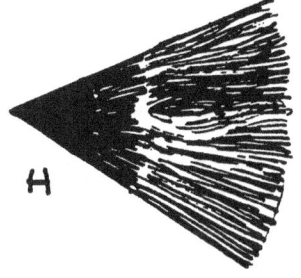

H

I — ROEMHELD SYNDROME:

INDICATED BY:
STRONG DILATION OF THE COLON ANW IN THE DIRECTION OF THE HEART AREA.

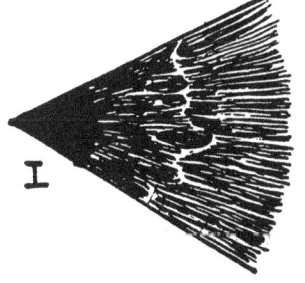

I

J — COLOURED FLECKS IN THE HEART AREA:
INDICATED BY: DISCOLORATIONS IN THE HEART AREA.
SYMPTOMS:
MENTAL DISTURBANCES
BROODING, MELANCHOLIC TENDENCIES
DEPRESSION
IT IS A RESULT OF TOXINS ACCUMULATION IN THE CIRCULATORY SYSTEM.

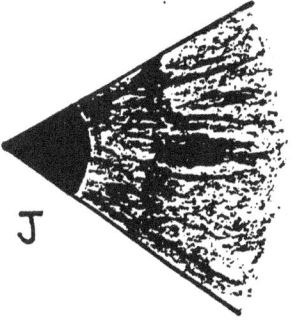

J

HEART CONDITIONS

WHOLISTIC APPROACH.

IT IS NOT THAT NECESSARILY TO DETECT THESE TEN CONDITIONS DURING IRIS READINGS OF PATIENTS
THE HEART IS A PART OF THE BODY, SO IT IS AFFECTED BY CONSTITUTION.
MANY CONDITIONS MAY HELP TO DETECT HEART CONDITIONS (WITHOUT FALLING INTO CONFUSION) SUCH AS:

1 _ GOOD CONSTITUTION (SILK IRIS), OR BAD CONSTITUTION (HESSIAN OR NET PATTERNS) INDICATE THE CONDITION OF THE WHOLE ORGANS, AND HELP THE PRACTICIONER TO FIND THE BALANCING FACTORS.
2 _ CONSTIPATION AND DILATION OF THE ANW INDICATE HEART TROUBLE
3 _ CHRONIC CONSTIPATION AND DIVERTICULI IN THE DESCENDING COLON, CAUSE HEART TROUBLE AND SEVER ATTACKS DUE TO THE GASES CONDITION.
4 _ SCURF RIM IN THE LOWER EXTREMETIES INDICATE AN OVER WORKING OR DIFFICULT PUMPING HEART.
5 _ ARCUS SENILIS INDICATE AN EXHAUSTED CONDITION OF THE HEART, BEING UN ABLE TO PUMP BLOOD TO THE HEAD AREA.
6 _ BRONCHITIS, ASTHMA & TUBERCULOSIS IRIS SIGNS, ALL CONTRIBUTE TO HEART FATIGUE.
7 _ LYMPHIC ROSARY INDICATE A CONDITION OF LYMPHIC CONGESTION AND CONTRIBUTE TO HEART FATIGUE AND TOXIC CIRCULATION.
8 _ TOXINS LADENED INTO LIVER, SPLEEN, KIDNEYS, LUNGS ALL CONTRIBUTE TO HEART MUSCLES WEAKNESS AND DIFFICULT PUMPING.
9 _ SODIUM RING, LEAD TO CORONARY SCLEROSIS CONDITION.

CAUSES:

BAD CONSTITUTION, INHERITED WEAKNESSES.
CONSTIPATION, AND ALL ITS CAUSES.
TOXICITY.
POLLUTION, DRUGS, TOBACO, ALCOHOLS, FATS, SUGARS.
STRESS, PLASTIC CIVILIZATION.
SEDATIVE LIFE STYLE, LACK OF EXERCISE.
MAGNESIUM DEFICIENCY.

TREATMENTS:

CLEANSING, PURIFICATIONS.
ELIMINATIONS.
VEGETABLES FASTINGS.
REST, MEDITATION, YOGA.
BREATHING & RELAXATION EXERCISE.
MULTI MINERALS / VITAMINS (FD)
BARE FEET WALKING ON EARTH
STRICT VEGAN DIET.

AVOID:

STRESS, EMOTIONS
ANXIETY
POLITICAL NEWS.
SUGARS, COFFEE, ALCOHOLS, FRIED FOODS, ROASTED SALTED NUTS, PEANUT BUTTER, ANIMAL FATS, VEGETARIAN HYDRO-GENATED FATS, BAD QUALITY OILS.

O HAEMORRHOIDS (PILES)

IRIS SIGNS:
DARK BOWELS AREA, DARK POCKETS.
DARK RECTUM AREA
BLACK SPOTS IN ANUS AREA.
SCURF RIM
DISCOLORATIONS IN GALL BLADDER
YELLOW_ORANGE_BROWN ANW.

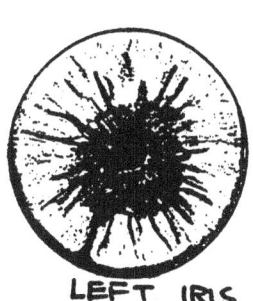

LEFT IRIS

INDICATIONS:
CONSTIPATION.
POOR BLOOD CIRCULATION IN LOWER EXTREMITIES
TOXIC GALL BLADDER CONDITION
TOXIC BLOOD SUPPLY.

CAUSES:
CONSTIPATION.
WHOLE FOOD DEFICIENCY.
OVER EATING.
POOR MUSCLES TONE.
HYPOFUNCTIONS OF LIVER & GALL BLADDER.
DEPENDING ON LAXATIVES.
POOR BLOOD CIRCULATION.

WHOLISTIC RELATIONSHIPS:
DIGESTIVE & CIRCULAR SYSTEMS
DIGESTIVE & MUSCULAR SYSTEMS
DIGESTIVE & NERVOUS SYSTEMS.

TREATMENTS:
TREAT CONSTIPATION.
LIVER FLUSH, GALL BLADDER CLEANSING.
WATER FASTING.
RECTAL BOWS   (FD)

O HEPATIC FLEXURE (SEE CHART PAGE H9)
O HEPATITIS (SEE LIVER CONDITIONS)
O HIGH BLOOD PRESSURE (SEE BLOOD PRESSURE)
O HYPERACTIVITY

IRIS SIGNS:
WHITENESS IN SENSORY LOCOMOTION AREA
WHITENESS IN OTHER IRIS AREAS.

INDICATES:
HYPERACTIVITY
ACIDITY
SPASM, PAIN.

RIGHT IRIS

CAUSES:
IMPROPER DIET
HYPERACIDITY
ACID ALKALINE IMBALANCE
HYPOFUNCTION OF ELIMINATIVE CHANNELS
MINERALS IMBALANCES.

HYPERACTIVITY

WHOLISTIC RELATION SHIPS:
  CIRCULATORY & NERVOUS SYSTEMS
  CIRCULATORY & DIGESTIVE SYSTEMS
  CIRCULATORY & ENDOCRINE SYSTEMS

TREATMENT:
  ELIMINATE ACIDITY
  ACID ALKALINE BALANCING
  STIMULATE ALL ELIMINATIVE CHANNELS
  PHYSICAL EXERCISE
  AVOID DAIRY PRODUCTS.

O HYPOGLYCEMIA (LOW BLOOD SUGAR)
  IRIS SIGNS:
  WEAK CONNECTIVE FIBERS.
  WHITE PANCREAS.
  BROWNISH ADRENALS.
  BROWN LIVER.
  WEAKNESS LESION THYROID.
  DARK BOWELS

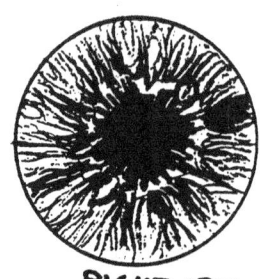

RIGHT IRIS

  INDICATIONS:
  POOR BODY TONE
  HYPERACTIVE PANCREAS
  ADRENAL EXHAUSTION
  LIVER CONGESTION
  HYPOTHYROIDISM
  CONSTIPATION

  CAUSES:
  PLASTIC LIFE STYLE.
  EXCESS REFINED CARBOHYDRATES.
  POOR PROTEIN ASSIMILATION.
  LACK OF FRESH VEGETABLES.
  ACID ALKALINE IMBALANCES.
  LACK OF PHYSICAL ACTIVITY.
  ENDOCRINE IMBALANCES
  ENDOCRINE HYPOFUNCTIONS
  DRUGS/POLLUTION
  MINERALS IMBALANCES

WHOLISTIC RELATION SHIPS:
  ALL SYSTEMS INVOLVED
TREATMENTS:
  BOWELS CLEANSING.
  LIVER, KIDNEYS/GALL BLADDER CLEANSING.
  HIGH PROTIEN DIET
  HIGH RAW FRESH VEGETABLES DIET
  WHOLE RICE, WHOLE WHEAT, RICH ZINC/SELENIUM/CHROMIUM.
AVOID: ALL FRUITS
       FATS
       STARCHES

○ HYSTERIA

IRIS SIGNS:
WHITENESS IN SEX IMPULSE AREA (RIGHT IRIS).
ACUTE NERVE RINGS IN BRAIN AREA.
DARK BOWELS AREA.
HETEROCHROMIA UPPER ANW.
WHITENESS IN SOLAR PLEXUS.
TIGHT ANW.
WHITENESS IN EQUILIBRIUM AREA (LEFT IRIS).
PSORIC SPOT IN ADRENAL GLAND.

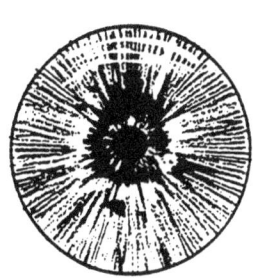

LEFT IRIS

INDICATIONS:
ACUTE BRAIN HYPERACTIVE CONDITION.
CONSTIPATION.
TRANSVERSE COLON IMPULSES INTO HEAD AREAS.
HYPER ACTIVE NERVOUS SYSTEM.
TENSION
TOXIC ADRENAL
PITUITARY & PENEAL GLANDS DIMINISHED FUNCTION
    CAUSED BY TRANSVERSE COLON CONDITION.

CAUSES:
ADRENAL IMBALANCE.
ENDOCRINE IMBALANCES.
CONSTIPATION & ALL ITS CAUSES.
INHERITED ACIDIC CONDITION.
STRESS.
ACID ALKALINE IMBALANCES.
POOR ELIMINATION.
STRESS-FUL OCCUPATION
LACK OF PHYSICAL EXERCISE
LACK OF DIRECT CONTACT WITH EARTH

WHOLISTIC RELATION SHIPS.
NERVOUS & ENDOCRINE SYSTEMS
NERVOUS & DIGESTIVE SYSTEMS
NERVOUS & CIRCULATORY SYSTEMS

TREATMENT,
BOWELS CLEANSING
ACID ALKALINE BALANCING
ALKALINE FORMULA (FD)
BLOOD PURIFYING   (FD)
BLOOD CIRCULATION (FD)
ENDOCRINE FORMULAS
NERVE TONIC
HYDROTHERAPIES
DIRECT CONTACT WITH EARTH.
REFLEXOLOGY, YOGA, ACUPUNCTURE.

CHART TO IRIDOLOGY

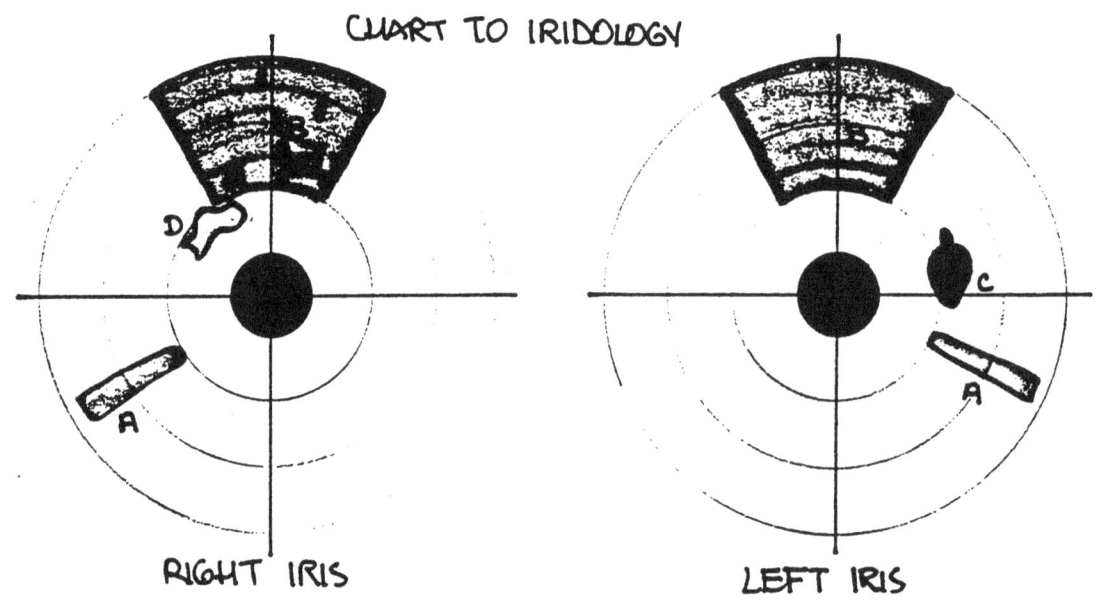

RIGHT IRIS   LEFT IRIS

A — HAND.
B — HEAD AREA.
C — HEART.
D — HEPATIC FLEXURE.

BASED ON CHARTS TO IRIDOLOGY DEVELOPED BY
Dr. BERNARD JENSEN & DOROTHY HALL

O ILEO-CECAL VALVE (SEE CHART PAGE I5)
O ILEO-CECAL VALVE CONDITIONS
   (SEE BOWELS CONDITIONS AND APPENDICITIS)

O IMMUNE SYSTEM

A— IRIS SIGNS:
   SILK IRIS FINE PATTERN
   TIGHT REGULAR ANW
   BRIGHTNESS, LIGHT

   INDICATIONS:
      GOOD CONSTITUTION
      RECOVER QUICKLY
      EXCELLENT IMMUNITY.

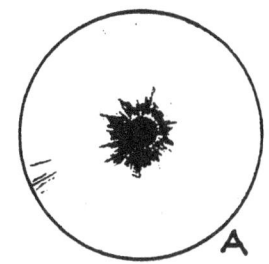 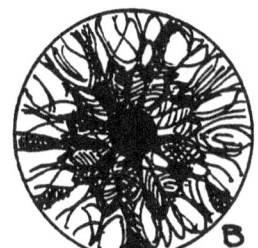

B— IRIS SIGNS:
   COARSE PATTERN
   WEAK CONNECTIVE TISSUE
   DILATED PUPIL
   DILATED FLOWER PATTERN ANW

   INDICATIONS:
      BAD CONSTITUTION
      SLOW HEALING PROCESS
      VERY BAD IMMUNITY.

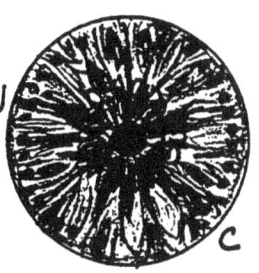 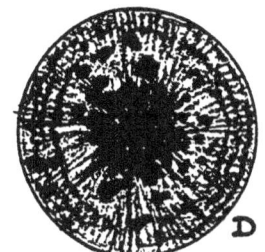

C— IRIS SIGNS:
   LYMPHIC ROSARY
   COARSE PATTERN
   DARKNESS SPLEEN AREA

   INDICATIONS:
      C VITAMIN DEFICIENCY
      BAD CONSTITUTION
      IMPAIRED IMMUNE SYSTEM CAUSED BY LYMPHIC
      CONGESTION & SPLEEN EXHAUSTION
      POOR DRAINAGE AND DIMINISHED FUNCTION OF
      ANTI BODIES.

D— IRIS SIGNS:
   GREEN IRIS
   PSORIC SPOTS
   NERVE RINGS

   INDICATIONS:
      DRUGS OVER USE
      VACCINATIONS
      IRRITATION
      IMPAIRED IMMUNE SYSTEM CAUSED BY DRUGS
      AND SUPPRESSIVE TREATMENTS.

BALANCING TREATMENTS:
   TREAT THE LYMPH SYSTEM (SEE LYMPH SYSTEM).
   ALL CLEANSING MEASURES.
   RICH SOURCES C, A & B VITAMINS (VEG. SOURCES).
   ALKALINE FORMULA (FD).
   MINERAL BALANCING.
   ENDOCRINE BALANCING.

O IMPOTENCE MALE

A_ IRIS SIGNS:
   ARCUS SINILES, SCURF RIM
   ANW DISCOLORATION.
   ANW DARKNESS CLOSE TO GENITO_URINARY
      AREA.
   DARK TESTES, PENIS AREAS.
   DARK ADRENALS
   DARK BOWELS

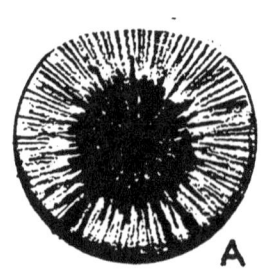

A

   INDICATIONS:
   DIMINISHED BRAIN QUALITY
   WEAK CEREBRAL FUNCTION
   TOXIC & CLOGGED BLOOD CIRCULATION
   CLOGGED BLOOD SUPPLY TO GENITO_URINARY AREA.
   INHERITED WEAKNESSES.
   ATROPHY IN SEXUAL ORGANS.
   CONSTIPATION, FAECES ACCUMULATIONS IN CECUM
      AND SIGMOID COLONS.

B_ IRIS SIGNS:
   DARKNESS IN BACK AREA.
   NERVE RINGS STARTING FROM PELVIC AREA TO TESTES
      AREA.
   INDICATIONS:
   POSTURE UN_ALIGNMENT.
   PELVIC LESIONS.
   IMPAIRED FUNCTION OF PELVIC NERVES.

B

OTHER CONDITIONS:
1_ RADII SOLERIS, INDICATE: TOXIC SEEPAGE INTO
      SEX ORGANS CAUSE DAMAGE AND
      DETERIORATION.
2_ TRANSVERSE COLON PROLAPSUS CAUSES A PERMANENT
      DAMAGE TO SEX ORGANS.
3_ SODIUM RING IN THE LOWER PART OF THE IRIS
      INDICATE HARDENING OF THE ARTERIES AND
      DIMINISHED BLOOD QUALITY TO SEX ORGANS.
4_ RADIALS FROM PUPIL TO SEX ORGANS INDICATE
      WEAKNESS OF CENTRAL NERVOUS SYSTEM.

CAUSES: DEPENDS UPON THE VARIOUS CONDITIONS AS
         OBSERVED IN THE IRIS.
WHOLISTIC RELATIONSHIPS:
      ALL SYSTEMS INVOLVED.
TREATMENT:
      DEPENDS UPON THE VARIOUS CAUSATIVE FACTORS
AND CONDITIONS AS ABOVE.
      YOU MAY REFER TO THE TREATMENTS OF THE
CONDITIONS IN MANY PAGES OF THIS DICTIONARY.

O INFECTIONS (SEE ACUTE STAGE OF DISEASE)
(SEE ACIDITY)
(SEE TONSILITIS)
(SEE APPENDICITIS)
(SEE BLADDER CONDITIONS)
(SEE KIDNEY CONDITIONS)
(SEE BRONCHITIS)
(SEE SINUSITIS)
(SEE GASTRITIS)
(SEE LIVER CONDITIONS)
(SEE PROSTATITIS)
(SEE LYMPHIC SYSTEM)
(SEE PEYER'S PATCHES)
(SEE THYMUS CONDITIONS)

O INFERTILITY FEMALE

A— ARCUS SENIUS, SCURF RIM
DARK BOWELS, PULLED ANW TOWARDS
IRIS RIM, DARK DAMAGED OVARY
AND UTERUS
INDICATE: INFERTILITY CAUSED BY
ANS, CIRCULATORY & DIGESTIVE SYSTEMS

B— DARK BACK (LUMBER AREA)
AND PELVIC AREA.
NERVE RINGS STARTING FROM PELVIS
TO OVARY AREA.
INDICATES: INFERTILITY CAUSED BY
NERVOUS & SKELETAL SYSTEMS

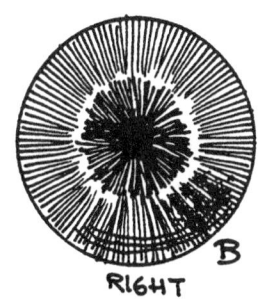
A RIGHT
B RIGHT

C— PULLED ANW TOWARDS PUPIL
TRANSVERSE COLON AREA
INDICATE: PROLAPSUS BOWEL
CONDITION CAUSING TEMPORY OR
PERMANENT OVARY DAMAGE.

D— RADIALS FROM PUPIL TO OVARY
INDICATE: INFERTILITY CAUSED BY
NERVOUS SYSTEM (CENTRAL NERVOUS
SYSTEM) CNS.

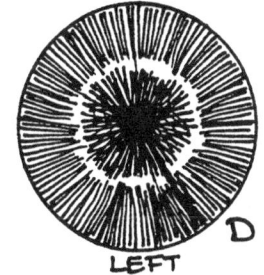
C
D LEFT

E— WEAKNESS LESION AND NERVE
RINGS PASS OVER THE OVARY
INDICATE: INHERED WEAKNESS
AND IRRITATION CAUSING THE
INFERTILITY CONDITION.

F— NERVE RINGS STARTING FROM
BRAIN AREA TO SEX ORGANS
INDICATE: INFERTILITY CAUSED BY
CEREBRAL IRRITATION.

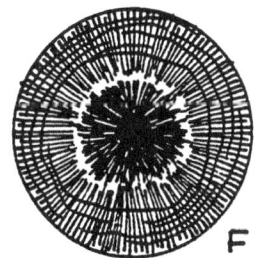
E
F

CAUSES: DEPEND UPON THE VARIOUS CONDITIONS AS OBSERVED
IN THE IRIS.
WHOLISTIC RELATION SHIPS:
ALL SYSTEMS INVOLVED.
TREATMENT:
DEPEND UPON THE VARIOUS CAUSATIVE FACTORS
AND CONDITIONS AS ABOVE.
TREAT THE CAUSATIVE FACTOR FIRST.

O INHERENT WEAKNESS
(SEE CHART PAGE I 5)

O INSOMNIA

A _ IRIS SIGNS:
   DARK LIVER IN RIGHT IRIS
   DARK SPLEEN IN LEFT IRIS
   CAUSE INSOMNIA CONDITION.
B _ WHITE SIGN IN INHERENT MENTAL AREA
   BROWN OR DARK BROWN ADRENAL
   WHITE NERVE RINGS.
   INDICATE: INSOMNIA.
C _ SODIUM RING
   INDICATE: HIGH SODIUM LEVEL IN THE BLOOD
   WEAK CALCIUM ABSORBTION
   CAUSE INSOMNIA.

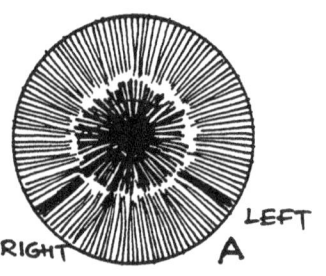

RIGHT   LEFT   A

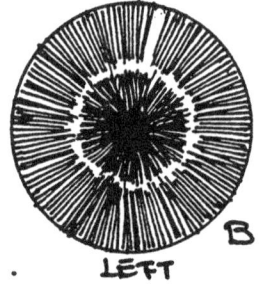

LEFT   B

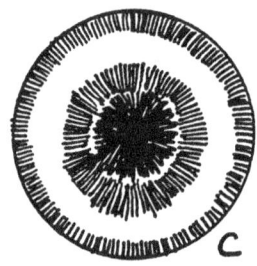

C

CAUSES:
   CONSTIPATION.
   EXCESS SODIUM, EXCESS DAIRY.
   POTASSIUM, CALCIUM & MAGNESIUM DEFICIENCY.
   B FAMILY VITAMINS DEFICIENCY
   C & E VITAMINS DEFICIENCY.
   HYPER OR HYPO-THYROIDISM.
   ADRENAL EXHAUSTION
   LIVER & SPLEEN CONGESTION
   ANEMIA
   ALCOHOLICS.
   INHERITED WEAK NERVOUS SYSTEM.
   EXHAUSTED PANCREAS.
   POOR BREATHING.

WHOLISTIC RELATION SHIPS:
   NERVOUS & CIRCULATORY SYSTEMS
   NERVOUS & DIGESTIVE SYSTEMS.
   NERVOUS & ENDOCRIN SYSTEMS
   NERVOUS & MUSCULAR SYSTEMS.

TREATMENTS:
   BOWELS CLEANSING, LIVER FLUSH, CASTOR OIL PACKS.
   ACID ALKALINE BALANCING.
   MULTI MINERALS / VITAMINS (FD)
   SWEET SLEEP FORMULA (FD)
   BLOOD PURIFICATION (FD)
   BLOOD CIRCULATION (FD)
   POTASSIUM BROTH
   RAW VEGETABLE BROTH
   EXERCISE / BREATHING EXERCISE
AVOID: SODIUM & IRON RICH FOODS.
   MEATS, DAIRY, EGGS, BREAD, SWEETS.
   COFFEE, TEA, ALCOHOLS.
   OVER DRINKING WATER
   WORK HARDLY AFTER SUN-SET

O INTUITION AREA
    (SEE CHART PAGE I5)

O INTESTINAL AREA
    (SEE DIGESTIVE SYSTEM CHART)

O INTESTINAL CONDITIONS
    (SEE BOWELS CONDITIONS)
    (SEE CONSTIPATION)

O INTESTINAL PARASITIS
    (SEE BOWELS CONDITIONS)

O IRRITATION
    (SEE NERVE RINGS)

CHART TO IRIDOLOGY

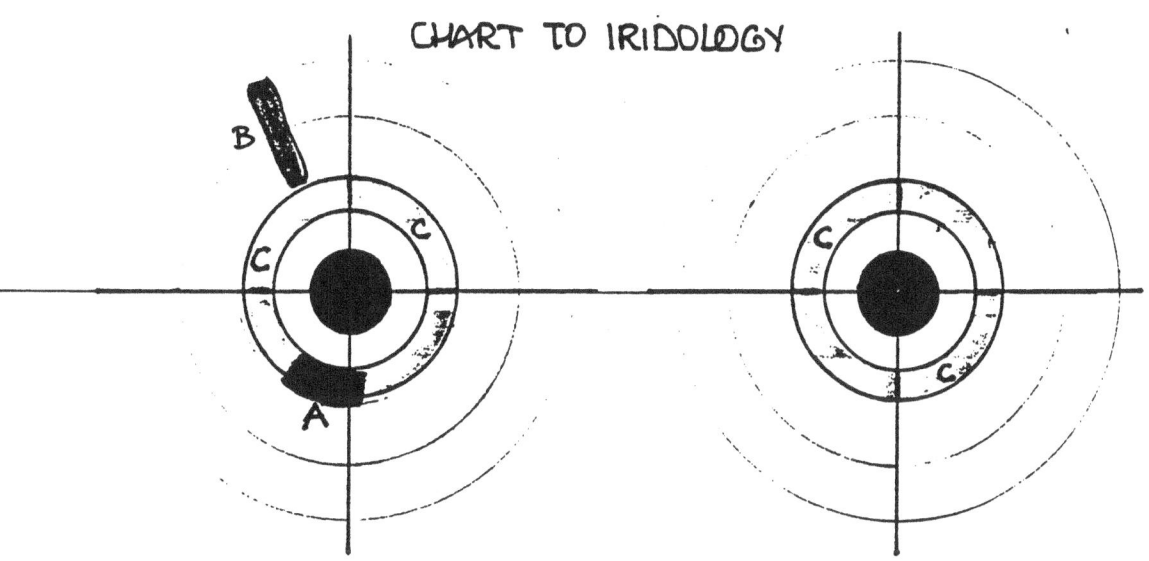

A— ILEO-CECAL VALVE
B— INTUITION (MENTAL ABILITY) AREA
C— INTESTINES AREA. (SEE ALSO DIGESTIVE SYSTEM)
D— INHERENT WEAKNESS

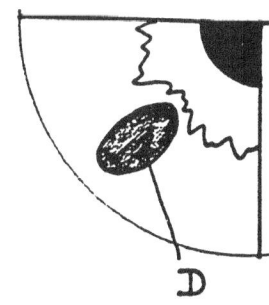

D

O JAUNDICE

IRIS SIGNS:

YELLOW SCLERA.
PSORIC SPOT IN LIVER AREA.
DISCOLORATION IN LIVER AREA.
YELLOW-ORANGE-BROWN ANW CLOSE
   TO GALL BLADDER & LIVER AREAS.
LYMPHIC ROSARY
NERVE RINGS
SCURF RIM

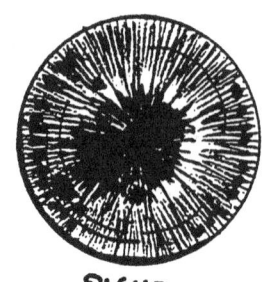

RIGHT

NOTE: THESE IRIS SIGNS MAY NEVER
   EXIST ALL TOGETHER AT ONE TIME.

INDICATIONS:

TOXIC CONDITION OF THE LIVER.
TOXIC BLOOD SUPPLY INTO LIVER.
LYMPHIC CONGESTION.
NERVOUS IRRITATION.
POOR BLOOD CIRCULATION

CAUSES:

FATS CONSUMPTION EXCESS.
OVER WORKING LIVER, LIVER EXHAUSTION.
TOXIC RETENTION INTO LIVER DUE TO
FAILURE FUNCTION OF BLOOD PURIFICATION
AND ELIMINATION.
TOXIC BLOOD SUPPLY TO LIVER DUE TO TOXIC
   BOWELS CONDITIONS.
SPLEEN HYPOFUNCTION.
LYMPHIC CONGESTION.
NDOCRINE IMBALANCES.
SPINAL LESIONS (THORACIC & CRANIAL)
METAL TOXICITY

WHOLISTIC RELATION SHIPS:

CIRCULATORY & DIGESTIVE SYSTEMS
CIRCULATORY & LYMPHIC SYSTEMS
CIRCULATORY & ELIMINATIVE CHANNELS.

TREATMENT:

BLOOD PURIFICATION (FD)
BLOOD CIRCULATION (FD)
ANEMIA FORMULA (FD)
RICH VEGETARIAN PROTIENS.
DRIED FRUITS
REST.
JAUNDICE FORMULA (FD) RESTORES LIVER TO
   NORMAL CONDITIONS.
CASTOR OIL PACKS
GALL BLADDER CLEANSING.
URINE THERAPY.

O KIDNEY AREA (SEE CHART PAGE K2)
O KIDNEY CONDITIONS

A_ IRIS SIGNS:
  KIDNEY MEDUSSA
  INDICATION:
    INTEGRATED DISFUNCTION
    OF THE KIDNEY & ADRENAL
    WITH INFLAMMATION.

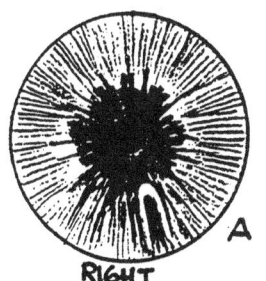

RIGHT

B_ WHITE OR PINK_RED RADIALS WITH
  DARK OPENINGS BETWEEN
  INDICATE:
    IRRITATION
    CHRONIC KIDNEY CONDITION.

C_ LYMPHATIC TOPHI IN KIDNEY
  AREA.
  INDICATES:
    TOXIC KIDNEY CONDITION

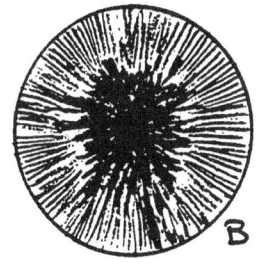

D_ NERVE RINGS STARTING FROM
  KIDNEY TO BACK AREA, AND PULLED TO KIDNEY AREA
  INDICATE:
    TROUBLES IN THE KIDNEY
    CAUSED BY AUTONOMIC NERVES
    IMPULSES.

E_ DARK RADII SOLERIS RADIATING FROM
  BOWEL AREA INTO KIDNEY AREA.
  INDICATE:
    TOXIC SEEPAGE FROM BOWELS INTO
    KIDNEY CAUSING BROWN & BAD SMELL OF THE
    URINE.

CAUSES:
  MEATS, DAIRY FOOD EXCESS.
  STARCHES, REFINED SUGARS EXCESS.
  CONSTIPATION.
  POOR CIRCULATION.
  POOR ELIMINATION.
  INHERITED WEAKNESS.
  NATURAL FLUIDS (VEG. SOURCES) DEFICIENCY.
  CALCIUM OXALATES RICH FOOD EXCESS
      SPINACH, CHOCOLETS, C VITAMIN
      SUPPLEMENTS EXCESS.
  DRUGS USE.
  SUPPRESSED TREATMENTS FOR VARIOUS
      INFECTIONS: THROAT, TONSILES.
  TOO MUCH WATER.
  STRESS, ADRENAL IMBALANCE.
  COFFEE, TEA, ALCOHOLS.

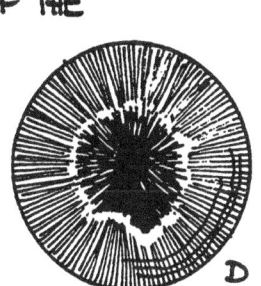

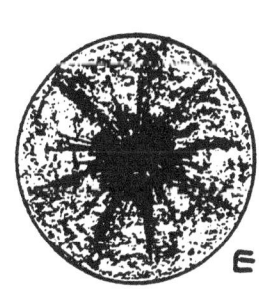

WHOLISTIC RELATIONSHIPS:
  URINARY & CIRCULATORY SYSTEMS
  URINARY & NERVOUS SYSTEMS
  URINARY & DIGESTIVE SYSTEMS
  URINARY & SKELETAL SYSTEMS.

KIDNEY CONDITIONS:

TREATMENTS:
VEGETABLE BROTH FAST
GRAPE FAST
POTASSIUM BROTH FAST
PARSLEY LEAF & ROOT TEA
BARELY
LICORICE
WATER MELLON SEED TEA
TREAT CONSTIPATION
TREAT BLOOD PURIFYING AND CIRCULATING.
ANTI-OBESE FORMULA (Dr.C)
KIDNEY BLADDER FORMULA (Dr.C)

K CHART

CHART TO IRIDOLOGY

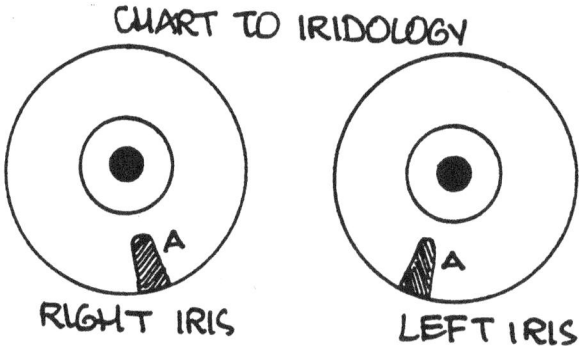

RIGHT IRIS   LEFT IRIS

A - KIDNEY   SEE ALSO URINARY SYSTEM.
              SEE ALSO ELIMINATIVE CHANNELS.
              SEE ALSO GENITO-URINARY AREA.

O LARYNX AREA (SEE CHART PAGE L4)
O LEG AREA (SEE CHART PAGE L4)
O LIVER AREA (SEE CHART PAGE L4)
O LIVER CONDITIONS

A _ IRIS SIGNS:
LYMPHIC ROSARY
WHITE _YELLOW RADIALS FROM DUODENUM
   AREA TO LIVER AREA
WHITE STREAKS IN LIVER AREA.
WHITE PEYER'S PATCHES.
YELLOW _ORANGE ANW.
INDICATIONS:
LYMPH CONGESTION
LIVER INFLAMMATION AND FEVER CAUSED
   BY TOXINS OVER LOAD IN THE BLOOD STREAM
   AND LIVER.
THIS CONDITION MAY EVENTUALLY LEAD TO
   HEPATITIS.

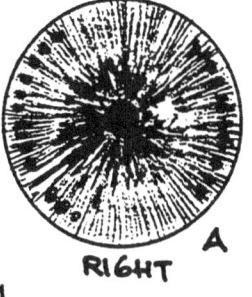

RIGHT   A

B _ IRIS SIGNS:
DARK BROWN LYMPHIC ROSARY
DARK BOWELS AREA.
SCURF RIM
DARK LIVER & GALL BLADDER AREAS

INDICATIONS:
SERIOUS CHRONIC LYMPHIC CONDITION
CONSTIPATION
VERY POOR BLOOD CIRCULATION
SERIOUS TOXIC LIVER CONDITION
LIVER IS IN A DEGENERATIVE STAGE.

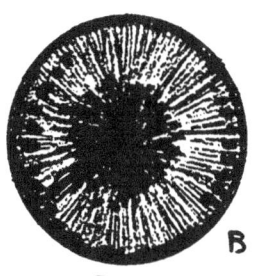

RIGHT   B

(SEE ALSO GALL BLADDER CONDITIONS)
(SEE ALSO JAUNDICE)

CAUSES:
CONSTIPATION AND ALL ITS CAUSES.
TOXICITY.
OVER LOADED LIVER (BY EXCESS FATS AND OILS)
   BEING UNABLE TO PURIFY BLOOD, LEAD EVENTUALLY
   TO HYPER FUNCTION AND CONGESTION.
LYMPHIC CONGESTION LOWERS THE IMMUNE SYSTEM
   LEAD TO TOXIC ACCUMULATION IN THE LIVER.
METAL POISONING
ANEMIA
POOR NUTRITION.

WHOLISTIC RELATION SHIPS:
DIGESTIVE & CIRCULATORY SYSTEMS
DIGESTIVE & LYMPHIC SYSTEMS
DIGESTIVE & ELIMINATIVE CHANNELS.

LIVER CONDITIONS

TREATMENT:
LIVER FLUSH
GALL BLADDER CLEANSING
TREAT CONSTIPATION
BOWELS CLEANSING
CASTOR OIL PACKS
LYMPHATIC FORMULA (FD)
LIVER GALL BLADDER FORMULA (FD)
ANEMIA FORMULA (FD)
BLOOD CIRCULATION (FD)
BLOOD PURIFICATION (FD)
DRIED FRUITS BROTH
ALMONDS, RAW FRESH VEGETABLES.
EXERCISE & REST

AVOID:
REFINED OILS
HYDROGENATED FATS
SATURATED FATS
FRIED FRUITS
REFINED SUGARS.
OVER EATING.
OVER SLEEPING.
ALCOHOLS, COFFEE, TEA, TOBACO.
EMOTIONAL STRESS.

O LOCOMOTION CENTER
    (SEE CHART PAGE L4)

O LUNGS AREA (SEE CHART PAGE L4)

O LUNGS CONDITIONS
    (SEE ASTHMA PAGE   )
    (SEE BRONCHITIS PAGE   )
(SEE ACIDITY PAGE   )
HYPER ACIDITY / WHITENESS IN THE IRIS:

INDICATE: A CATARRHAL CONDITION IN THE LUNGS
        AND MUCUS ACCUMULATION.
(SEE CANCER IN THE LUNG PAGE C2)
(SEE CANCER PAGE C2 IRIS B. THE SAME IRIS
    READING MAY INDICATE TUBERCULOSIS).

O LYMPHATIC SYSTEM CHART

CHART TO IRIDOLOGY

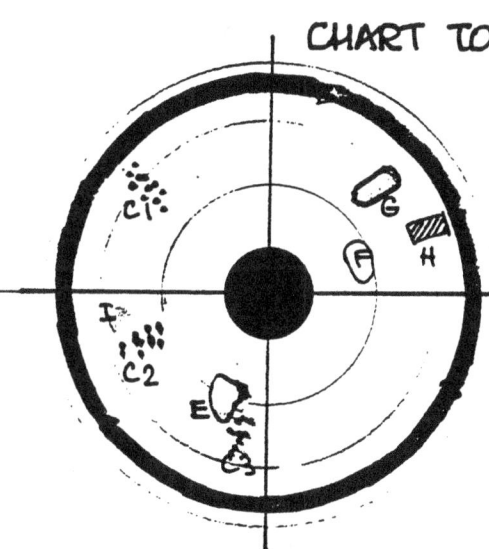

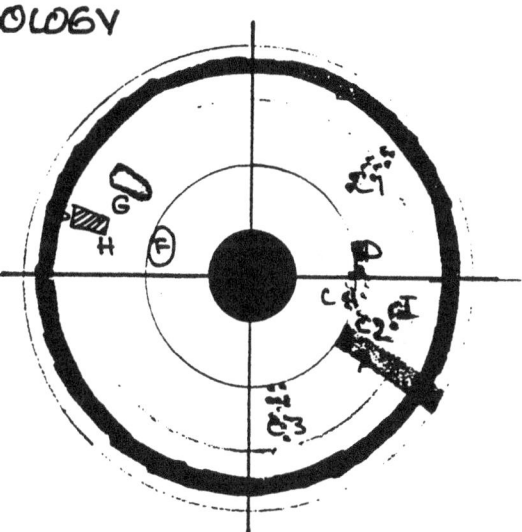

RIGHT IRIS	LEFT IRIS
A _ SPLEEN	D _ THYMUS GLAND
B _ LYMPHATIC ZONE	E _ APPENDIX
C _ LYMPH GLANDS	F _ PEYER'S PATCHES
C1 _ CERVICAL	G _ NOSE (ADENOIDS)
C2 _ AXILLA	H _ TONSILS
C3 _ GROIN	I _ MAMMARY GLANDS.
C4 _ SOLAR PLEXUS	

O LYMPHIC SYSTEM CONDITIONS

A _ IRIS SIGNS:
LYMPHATIC ROSARY
INDICATE: LYMPH CONGESTION CONDITION.
THE DARKER THE ROSARY, THE MORE
SERIOUS THE CONDITION.

B _ IRIS SIGNS:
BLUE IRIS LYMPHATIC TYPE.
INDICATE:
TENDENCY TO ARTHRITIS & RHEUMATISM.

TREATMENT OF LYMPH SYSTEM:
VIGORIOUS EXERCISE.
WALKING BARE FEET ON SAND OR GRASS.
SKIN BRUSHING, CASTOR OIL PACKS.
ALKALINE FORMULA (FD).
LYMPHATIC FORMULA (FD).
POTASSIUM BROTH, VEG. BROTH.
APPLE CIDER VINAGAR.
STIMULATE SKIN FUNCTION.
STRICT VEGAN DIET.
BLOOD CIRCULATION FORMULA (FD).
SUN BATHING, AIR BATHING, VENTILATION.
SWIMMING.

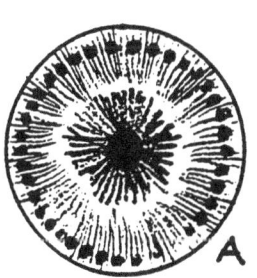

A

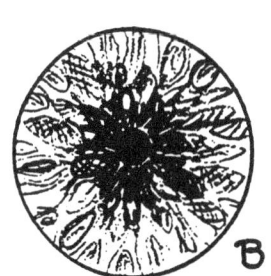

B

CHART TO IRIDOLOGY

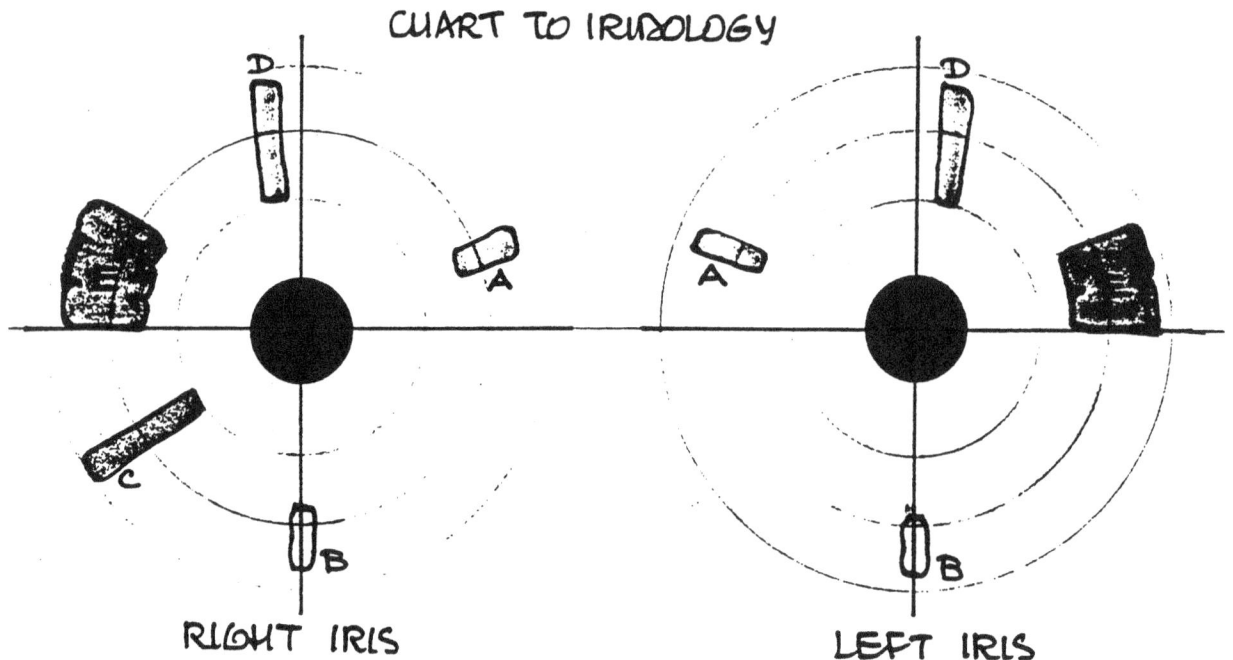

RIGHT IRIS   LEFT IRIS

A _ LARYNX
B _ LEG
C _ LIVER
D _ LOCOMOTION AREA
E _ LUNGS

○ MAMMARY GLANDS
(SEE CHART PAGE M7)
○ MAMMARY GLANDS CONDITIONS

A_ IRIS SIGNS:
WHITENESS IN MAMMARY GLAND AREA
INDICATE:
A HEALTHY CONDITION OF BREAST FEEDING.
TEMPORARY OVER FUNCTIONING OF THE
    BREAST DURING LACTATION.
OVARY AREA MAY ALSO WHITENED DUE
    TO OVARIAN HORMONE SECRETION
    (OESTROGEN)

RIGHT

B_ IRIS SIGNS:
PSORIC SPOT MAM. AREA.
NERVE RINGS PASSING THROUGH MAM. AREA.
LYMPHIC ROSARY
DARKNESS
SCURF RIM.
INDICATE:
BREAST CANCER CONDITION (TENDENCY)

CAUSES OF BREAST DISEASES:
DELAYED MARRIAGE & DELAYED LACTATION.
ANTI_LACTATIVE DRUGS.
BIRTH CONTROL PILLS.
LYMPHIC CONGESTION.
IRREGULAR MENSTRUATION.
DAIRY, MEATS, EGGS.
HIGH ACIDIC DIET.
LACK OF FRESH FRUITS & VEGETABLES.
BLOOD TOXICITY.
SUPPRESSED INFLAMMATIONS

WHOLISTIC RELATIONSHIPS:
LYMPHIC & CIRCULATORY SYSTEMS.
LYMPHIC & REPRODUCTIVE SYSTEMS.
LYMPHIC & DIGESTIVE SYSTEMS.
LYMPHIC & ENDOCRINE SYSTEMS.

TREATMENTS:
WATER FASTING
VEGETABLES JUICE FASTINGS / VEG. BROTH.
TREAT LYMPHATIC SYSTEM
BLOOD CIRCULATION & PURIFICATION
REST, MEDITATION.
STRICT LEAFY VEGETABLES DIET.
VEGAN DIET AFTER RECOVERY.

O MASTOID (SEE CHART PAGE M7)
O MEDULLA (SEE CHART PAGE M7)
O MEDULLA CONDITIONS

   IRIS SIGNS:

LEFT

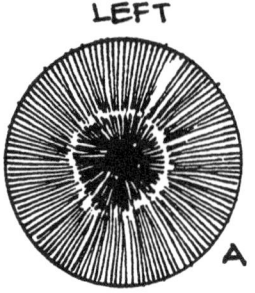

A _ WHITE SIGNS IN MEDULLA AREA.
   INDICATE:
   WELL CONTROLLED INDIVIDUAL
B _ YELLOW-BROWN SIGNS
   INDICATE:
   MEDULLA HYPOFUNCTION
   POOR NERVOUS RELATION BETWEEN
     BRAIN AND BODY.
   BREATHING TROUBLES.
C _ RADIALS FROM PUPIL TO MEDULLA.
   INDICATE:
   HYPOFUNCTION OF THE MEDULLA CAUSED
     BY TOXINS SEEPAGE FROM BOWELS
     VIA LYMPH CHANNELS & CIRCULATION.

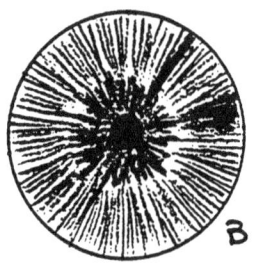

   CAUSES OF MEDULLA TROUBLES:

   POOR POSTURE.
   CERVICAL LESIONS.
   FAECES ACCUMULATION IN THE
     HEPATIC & SPLENIC FLEXURES.
   CONSTIPATION.
   INHERITED WEAKNESS.

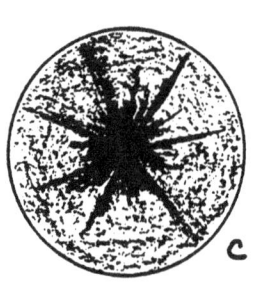

   WHOLISTIC RELATIONSHIPS:
   NERVOUS & RESPIRATORY SYSTEMS
   NERVOUS & CIRCULATORY SYSTEMS
   NERVOUS & SKELETAL SYSTEMS
   NERVOUS & LYMPHATIC SYSTEMS

   TREATMENT:
   TREAT CONSTIPATION (IF IT IS THE CAUSE)
   ALEXANDER TECHNIQUE
   CHIROPRACTICE
   BLOOD PURIFICATION (FD)
   NERVE TONIC (DrC)
   NERVE REJUVENATION (FJD)

O MENSTRUAL DISORDERS

   IRIS SIGNS:

1 _ BROWN OR LYMPHIC TOPHI IN OVARIAN AREA
   INDICATE: TOXIC OR WEAKENED FUNCTION OF OVARY
     CAUSING MENSTRUAL DISORDER.
2 _ BALLOONED BOWELS & POCKETS IN THE SIGMOID AND
   DESCENDING COLON.
   INDICATE: A CHRONIC CONSTIPATION CONDITION AFFECTING
     THE OVARIAN FUNCTION CAUSING MENSTRUAL DISORDERS.
     (SEE BOWELS CONDITIONS)

MENSTRUAL DISORDERS

3 _ THYROID, MAMMARY GLANDS & OVARIAN AREAS
DISCOLORATIONS
INDICATE: MENSTRUAL DISORDERS CAUSED BY ENDOCRINE
AND LYMPHATIC WEAKNESSES.
4 _ WHITE LINES IN THE UTERUS AREA.
INDICATE: OVER ACTIVITY AND MENSTRUAL PERIODS
OCCUR TOO FREQUENTLY.
MENSTRUAL DISORDER WITH PAIN.
5 _ DILATED ANW.
NERVE RINGS IN OVARIAN & UTERUS ARES.
INDICATE: MENSTRUAL DISORDERS CAUSED BY
ANS DISORDERS.
6 _ SODIUM RING
INDICATE: IN EARLY AGES
MENSTRUAL DISORDERS CAUSED BY CIRCULATION
TROUBLES.

CAUSES:
CHECK THE VARIOUS WHOLISTIC RELATION SHIPS
AS ABOVE AND MANY OTHERS.
WHOLISTIC RELATION SHIPS,
ALL SYSTEMS INVOLVED

TREATMENTS:
DEPENDS UPON: CAUSES
IRIS CONSTITUTION / IRIS TYPE.
WEAKNESS LESIONS AREAS
START & END OF NERVE RINGS.
WHOLISTIC RELATION SHIPS.

O MENTAL ABILITY
(SEE CHART PAGE   )

O METABOLISM CONDITIONS
A _ IRIS SIGNS:
WHITENESS
INDICATE:
HYPER ACIDITY
TENDENCY TO ARTHRITIS & RHEUMATISM
INCREASED METABOLIC PROCESS.

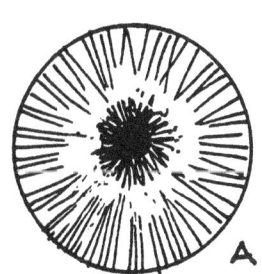

B _ IRIS SIGNS:
SCURF RIM
INDICATE:
TOXIC & POOR CIRCULATION
UNDER FUNCTION OF SKIN
LOW METABOLIC RATE.

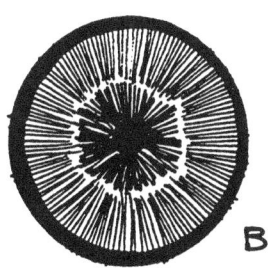

METABOLIC DISORDERS.

C — IRIS SIGNS:
   DARK THYROID AREA.
   INDICATION:
   HYPOTHYROIDISM.
   LOW METABOLIC RATE.

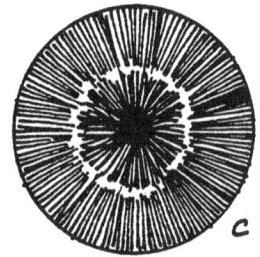

D — DARK STOMACH RING
   INDICATION:
   UNDER ACID STOMACH
   LOW METABOLIC FUNCTION.

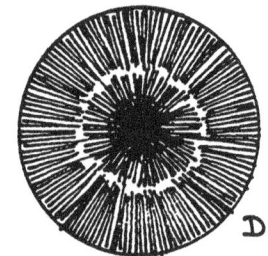

CAUSES:
   HYPER ACIDITY
   ACID ALKALINE IMBALANCES
   CONSTIPATION
   BLOOD QUALITY
   CONSTITUTIONAL TYPE.
   POOR ELIMINATION
   SODIUM/CALCIUM, HCL DEFICIENCIES.
   INTESTINAL PARASITIS
   LYMPH CONGESTION, ENDOCRINE IMBALANCES.

WHOLISTIC RELATION SHIPS
   DIGESTIVE & CIRCULATORY SYSTEMS.
   DIGESTIVE & ENDOCRINE SYSTEMS.
   DIGESTIVE & LYMPHIC SYSTEMS.

TREATMENT:
   ALKALINE FORMULA (FD)
   BLOOD PURIFYING (FD)
   BLOOD CIRCULATION (FD)
   KELP
   POTASSIUM BROTH
   FRESH FRUITS & VEGETABLES
   PANCREAS FORMULA (FD)
   EXERCISE

AVOID:
   DRINKING WITH MEALS
   CARBONATED BEVERAGES
   MIXING STARCH & PROTIENS IN ONE MEAL
   TABLE SALTS.

O MIGRAINE

IRIS SIGNS:

MIGRAINE HAS NO SPECIAL SIGNS IN THE IRIS
THE PATIENT WILL TELL YOU ABOUT HIS OR HER
MIGRAINE, SEVERITY AND WHICH SIDE OF THE HEAD.
CHECK IN THE IRIS THE CAUSATIVE FACTORS BY READING
THE FOLLOWING VERY IMPORTANT AREAS:

1 _ TRANSVERSE COLON CONDITIONS:
  a-PULLED TOWARDS UPPER IRIS RIM
  b.HETEROCHROMIA
  c-DISCOLORATIONS IN SINUS AREA.
  d_CLOGGED VENOUS SUPPLY TO HEAD INDICATED BY
    RADIALS FROM TRANSVERSE COLON AREA TO
    HEAD AREA AT 7' & 53' BOTH IRISES.
    (SEE CIRCULATORY SYSTEM CHART)
  e_DARKNESS OF THE TRANSVERS COLON, POCKETS.
  f_PROLAPSUS OF THE TRANSVERS COLON.

2 _ LIVER CONDITIONS:
  a_ LIVER AREA WEAKNESS LESION
  b_ PSORIC SPOT
  c_ RADIALS PASSING INTO LIVER, GALL BLADDER AND
    DUODENUM.
  d_ NERVE RINGS.
  e_ STAGE OF DISEASE

3 _ ENDOCRINE SYSTEM:
  a_ HYPO OR HYPERTHYROIDISM.
  b_ ADRENAL / INHERENT MENTAL AREAS AND THEIR
    RELATION WITH STRESS.

4 _ NERVOUS IRRITATION:
  a_ NERVE RINGS / START & END.

5 _ CIRCULATORY DISORDERS:
  a_ SCURF RIM IN HEAD AREA.
  b_ EGO PRESSURE AREA.
  c_ EXTREMETIES ANEMIA.
  d_ COLOUR OF THE ANW.

6 _ REPRODUCTIVE DISORDERS:
  a_ SEX IMPULSE / VAGINA, SEXUAL FRUSTRATION
  b_ MENSTRUAL DISORDERS.

7 _ RESPIRATORY DISORDERS:
  a_ LUNGS CONDITIONS.
  b_ MEDULLA.
  c_ BRONCHUS & BRONCHIALS.
  d_ STAGES OF DISEASE.
  e_ SKIN CONDITION.

TREATMENT:
  DEPENDS UPON THE ORGANS CONDITIONS INVOLVED
AS A CAUSATIVE FACTOR.

O MINERALS DEFICIENCIES

1 — CALCIUM DEFICIENCY
   IRIS SIGNS:
   DARKNESS IN SKELETAL AREAS

2 — CALCIUM IMBALANCE
   IRIS SIGNS:
   SODIUM RING
   WHITENESS OF THE ANW

3 — IODINE DEFICIENCY
   IRIS SIGNS:
   DARK THYROID AREA.

4 — IRON DEFICIENCY
   IRIS SIGNS:
   EXTREMETIES ANEMIA
   ANEMIA AT BRAIN
   ANEMIA RING

5 — MAGNESIUM DEFICIENCY.
   IRIS SIGNS:
   DARK EGO PRESSURE AREA.
   SODIUM RING
   IRIS WHITENESS (ACIDITY)
   LYMPHATIC ROSARY.

6 — PHOSPHOROUS IMBALANCES
   IRIS SIGNS:
   THICK WHITE ANW

7 — POTASSIUM DEFICIENCY
   IRIS SIGNS:
   THICK WHITE ANW, WHITENESS OF IRIS RIM.
   LYMPHATIC ROSARY
   WHITE STOMACH RING (STOMACH HYPERACIDITY)

8 — SODIUM DEFICIENCY
   IRIS SIGNS:
   DARK STOMACH RING (HYPOACID STOMACH)
   LYMPHIC ROSARY
   THICK WHITE ANW

9 — ZINC DEFICIENCY.
   IRIS SIGNS:
   DARK PROSTATE AREA
   DARK PANCREAS AREA.
   POOR CONNECTIVE FIBERS.

O MOUTH AREA (SEE CHART PAGE M7)

O MUCUS SETTELMENTS
   (SEE ACIDITY CONDITIONS)
   CAUSES AND TREATMENT:
   (SEE ACIDITY)

O MUSCLES AREA (SEE CHART PAGE M7)

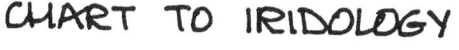

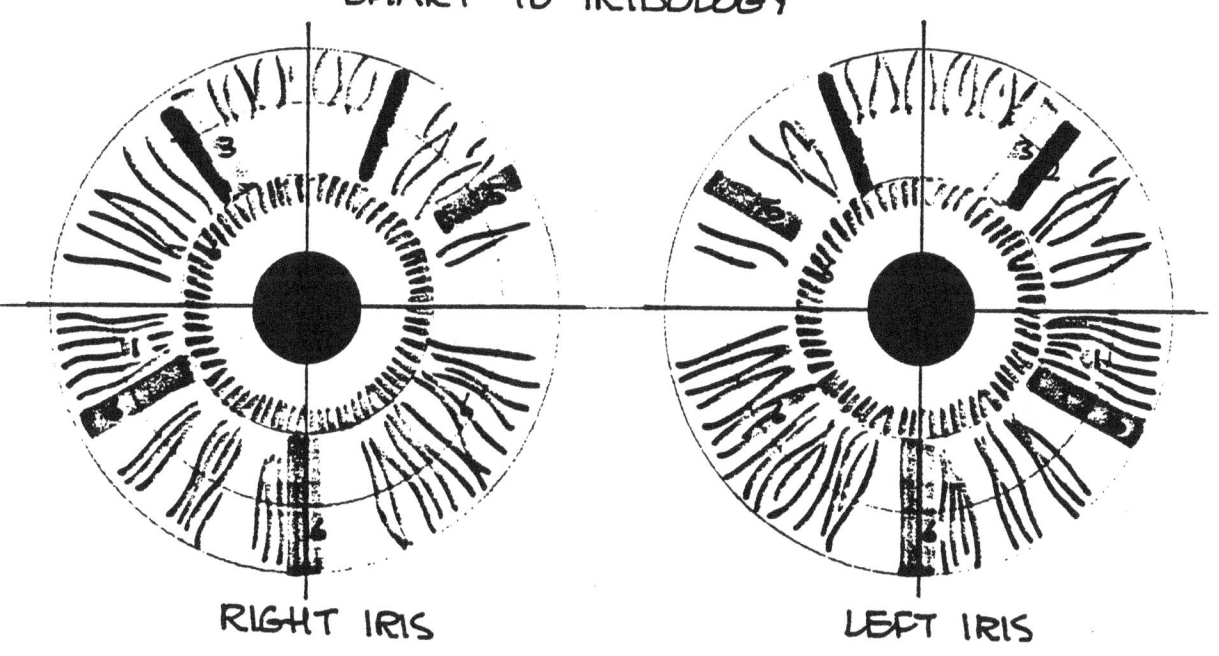

RIGHT IRIS   LEFT IRIS

1 _ MAMMARY GLANDS.
2 _ MASTOID
3 _ MEDULLA
4 _ MENTAL ABILITY
5 _ MOUTH
6 _ MUSCLES AREAS.

O NECK AREA (SEE CHART PAGE C4)
O NECK CONDITIONS (SEE SKELETAL SYSTEM)
O NERVOUS SYSTEM AREAS

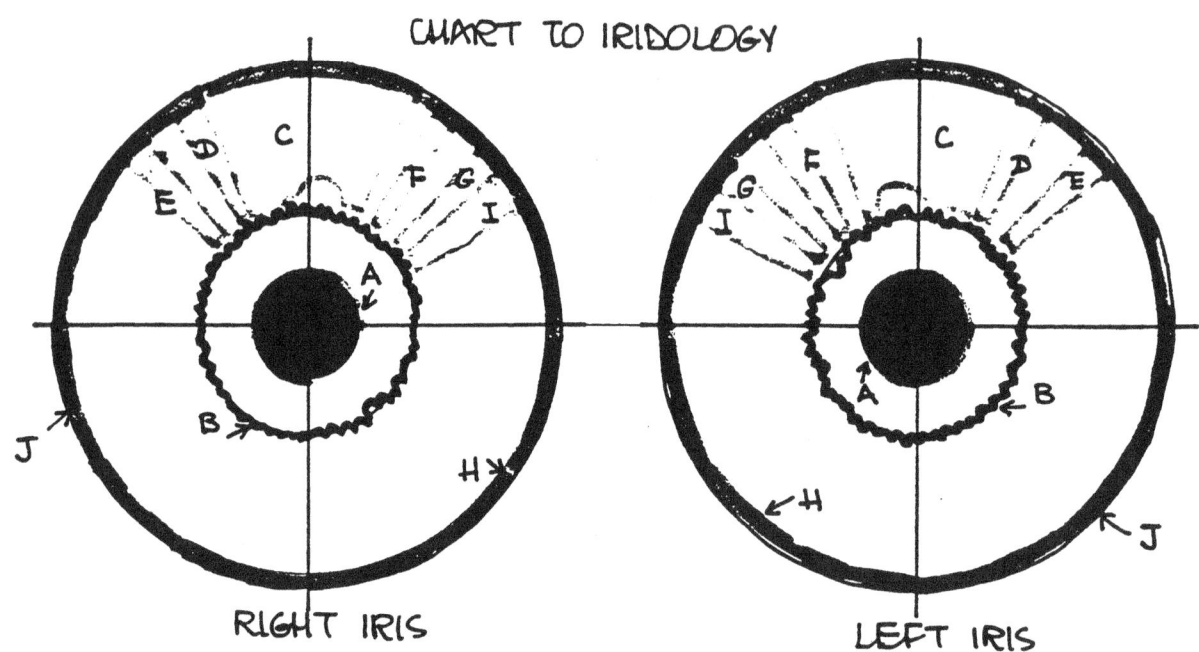

CHART TO IRIDOLOGY

RIGHT IRIS   LEFT IRIS

A — CENTRAL NERVOUS SYSTEM. CNS.
B — AUTONOMIC NERVOUS SYSTEM. ANS.
C — BRAIN AREA
D — MEDULLA
E — EAR
F — EYE
G — NOSE
H — SKIN
I — TONGUE
J — PARASYMPATHETIC NERVOUS SYSTEM. PNS.

O NERVOUS SYSTEM CONDITIONS
   (SEE AUTONOMIC NERVOUS SYSTEM PAGE A12)
   (SEE CENTRAL NERVOUS SYSTEM PAGE C3)

O NERVE RINGS

IRIS SIGNS:
CONTRACTIONS IN IRIS TISSUES
INDICATE:
MENTAL STRESS, PHYSICAL TENSION
SHOCKS, IRRITATION, TOXICITY
HYPER OR HYPOFUNCTION.

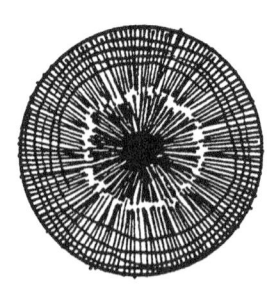

NERVE RINGS

CAUSES:

IRRITATION, DRUGS, STRESS, MALNUTRITION
LACK OF EXERCISE, BAD POSTURE
ANXIETIES, FRUSTRATIONS, POOR METABOLISM.

WHOLISTIC RELATION SHIPS:
NERVOUS SYSTEM & ALL SYSTEMS

TREATMENT OF NERVOUS SYSTEM:
1- CONTACT WITH EARTH:
     BARE FEET AND NAKED BODY WALKING ON
     SAND OR GRASS.
     SWIMMING, SLEEPING ON GRASS.
     BE FAR AWAY FROM PLASTIC CIVILIZATION.
     MEDITATION, MASSAGE, REFLEXOLOGY.
     YOGA, BREATHING EXERCISE.
2- DIET:
     LETTUCE, CAMMOMILE
     STRICT VEGAN DIET, MACROBIOTIC DIET.
  AVOID: MEATS, DARY, FISH, EGGS.
          COFFEE, TEA, ALCOHOLOS
          REFINED CARBOHYDRATES.

3- HERBAL:
     SWEET SLEEP FORMULA (PD)
     NERVE TONIC (DrC)
     NERVE REJUVENATION (FJD)

O OVARY AREA

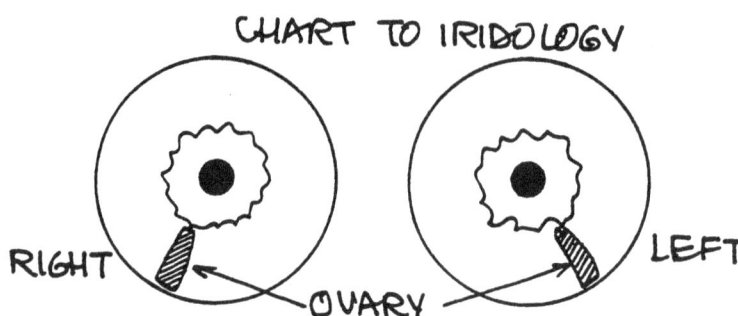

CHART TO IRIDOLOGY

RIGHT — OVARY — LEFT

O OVARY CONDITIONS

A — IRIS SIGNS:
   WHITE OVARY , WHITE OPPOSITE
      IN BRAIN AREA.
   INDICATE :
   DISTURBANCE IN SEXUAL LIFE .
   DEPRESSION.
   OPPRESSION.

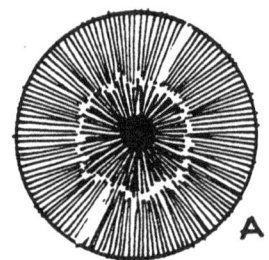
A

RIGHT

B — DARK OVARIAN AREA.
   PULLED ANW TOWARDS PUPIL
   INDICATE :
   PREMATURE MENOPAUSE.
   OVARIAN TUMOR .

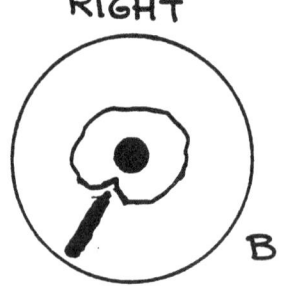
B

C — DISCOLORATION IN THYROID
      MAMMARY GLANDS & OVARIAN
      AREA.
   INDICATE :
   MENSTRUAL DISORDERS

NOTE: SEE ALSO MENSTRUAL DISORDERS
   (PAGE M2 — M3)

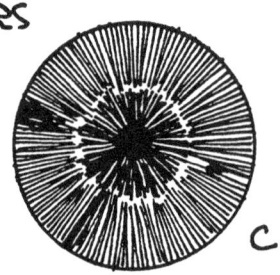
C

TREATMENT:
   BLOOD PURIFICATION
   BLOOD CIRCULATION
   VEGETABLE BROTH FAST
   BOWELS CLEANSING
   ALKALINE FORMULA
   NERVOUS SYSTEM TREATMENTS
   ENDOCRINE SYSTEM TREATMENT
   NERVE REJUVINATION
   REFLEXOLOGY
   ACUPUNCTURE
   CHIROPRACTICE (SPINAL CAUSES)

O OXYGEN DEFICIENCY

IRIS SIGNS:

1_ ANEMIA CONDITIONS (SEE ANEMIA: AT BRAIN EXTREMETIES, AND ANEMIA RING.

2_ FIBER PATTERNS OF IRIS:
SILK OR SILK_LINEN IRIS REVEAL THE CONSTITUTION CONDITION OF THE BODY. WHICH INDICATE THE STRENGTH AND GOOD LUNGS. THEY ALSO INDICATE A GOOD OXYGEN INTAKE

3_ COARSE FIBERS PATTERNS:
INDICATE:
POOR BODY TONE
WEAK MUSCULAR ABILITY
SMALL LUNGS, POOR BREATHING
OXYGEN DEFICIENCY.

4_ COARSE FIBERS PATTERNS WITH BLACK OPENINGS BETWEEN FIBERS. ADHESIONS.
INDICATE:
FREE RADICALS IMBALANCE, E VITAMIN DEFICIENCY
B FAMILY DEFICIENCY
COLLAGEN DEFICIENCY
SCURVY
OXYGEN STARVATION. TENDENCY TO CANCER.

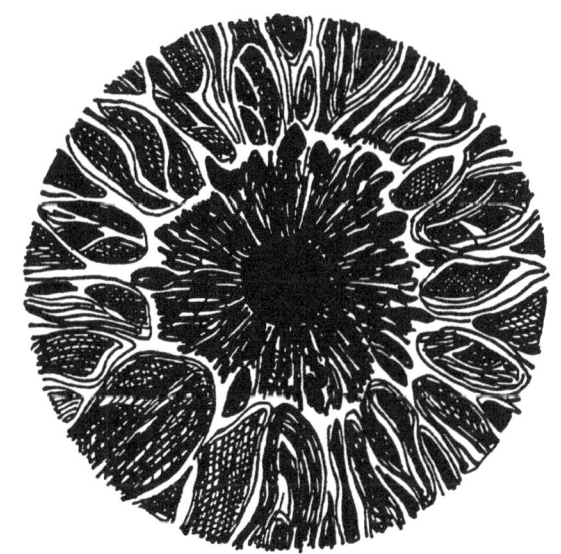

TREATMENT:
E VITAMIN, B FAMILY VITAMINS C VITAMIN
BIO-CHEMIC TISSUE SALTS
TREAT RESPIRATORY SYSTEM, TREAT MEDULLA
TREAT ANEMIA
TREAT INSOMNIA / DEPRESSION
TREAT NERVOUS SYSTEM.
CLEANSING PROGRAMMS
PURIFICATION PROGRAMMS.

O PANCREAS AREA (SEE CHART PAGE   )
O PANCREATIC CONDITIONS
      (SEE DIABETES PAGE   )
      (SEE HYPOGLYCEMIA PAGE   )

O PARASITIS INTESTINAL
  IRIS SIGNS:
  1_ SMALL BLACK SPOTS IN BOWELS
      AREA.
  2_ LYMPHIC TOPHI & ORANG_BROWN
      CLOUDS COVERING THE IRIS FIBERS
      IN THE INTESTINAL AREA.
  3_ SMALL BLACK LINES RADIATING
      FROM ANW INTO BODY ORGANS
      AREA

  INDICATIONS:
  1_ INTESTINAL PARASITIS DEVELOPED
      IN THE AREA AS IRIS REVEALS.
  2_ TOXIC BOWELS CONDITION CAUSED
      BY INTESTINAL PARASITIS.
  3_ DAMAGE (CAUSED BY A CHRONIC
      CONDITION OF INTESTINAL PARASITIS
      COLONIES) OF THE INTESTINAL WALL
      LEAD TO TOXIC SEEPAGE INTO VARIOUS
      BODY ORGANS.

  CAUSES:
    CONSTIPATION, CONTAMINATED FOOD, RAW MEATS
    UN-CLEANED RAW VEGETABLES
    BRAN & FIBER DEFICIENCY WHICH CAUSE CONSTIPATION
      ALLOW THE EGGS OF THE WORM TO GROW
      PEACEFULLY
    MEATS, EGGS & DAIRY ARE THE FAVOURITE NUTRIENT
      OF WORMS.
  WHOLISTIC RELATION SHIPS
  DIGESTIVE & RESPIRATORY SYSTEMS
  DIGESTIVE & CIRCULATORY SYSTEMS

  TREATMENT:
  GARLIC & ONION FAST
  PUMPKIN SEED FAST.
  FOLLOW BY HERBAL LAXATIVE
  EVACUATE IN A WARM MILK DEEP DISH, BY CONTACT
    DIRECTLY TO ANUS.

  IMPORTANT NOTE:
    WHEN A PARASITIS CONDITION OCCURE, READ
    CAREFULLY THE LUNGS, MEDULLA, ARCUS SENILIS
    AND CIRCULATORY CONDITIONS.

O PELVIC AREA (SEE CHART PAGE P5)

O PERSPIRATION

IRIS SIGNS:

1— SCURF RIM (SEE SCURF RIM PAGE S1)
INDICATE:
SUPPRESSE PERSPIRATION CONDITION BY THICK
UN_NATURAL CLOTHES, OR VERY POOR BODY
VENTILATION OR POOR SKIN BRUSHING AND
BATHING.

2— LYMPHATIC ROSARY (SEE LYMPHATIC ROSARY PAGE   )
INDICATE:
CLOGGED PERSPIRATION CONDITION CAUSED BY
NUTRITIONAL IMBALANCES AND LACK OF PHYSICAL
EXERCISE.

3— ANEMIA AT EXTREMETIES (SEE ANEMIA PAGE   )
INDICATE:
POOR FLUIDS SUPPLY TO SKIN AND COLD EXTREMETIES
CAUSING SKIN PORES CONTRACTION.

CAUSES:
RECINED CARBOHYDRATES.
MEATS, DAIRY, EGGS, FISH
POOR CONTACT WITH EARTH.
POOR BODY VENTILATION.
POTASSIUM, SODIUM, MAGNESIUM, IRON, IODINE
AND SILICON DEFICIENCIES.
LACK OF PHYSICAL EXERCISE
PERMANANT OPERATION OF AIR_COOLING SYSTEMS.
CONSTIPATION
STRESS, TENSION.
HUMID OCCUPATION

WHOLISTIC RELATION SHIPS:
RESPIRATORY & CIRCULATORY SYSTEMS
RESPIRATORY & LYMPHIC SYSTEMS
RESPIRATORY & URINARY SYSTEMS
RESPIRATORY & DIGESTIVE SYSTEMS

TREATMENT:
CONTACT WITH EARTH:
NAKED BODY MASSAGE ON SAND OR GRASS
BARE FOOT WALKING / SAND / GRASS
EXPOSE NAKED BODY TO NATURAL CLIMATE CONDITIONS.
AIR / SUN BATHING, SWIMMING, SAUNAS.
LYMPHATIC SYSTEM CLEANSING.
BREATHING EXERCISE.
ALKALINE ACID BALANCING
BOWELS CLEANSING
SKIN BRUSHING
FENUGREEK HERB TO STIMULATE SKIN FUNCTION.
STIMULATE ALL ELIMINATIVE CHANNELS.

O PEYER'S PATCHES (SEE CHART PAGE P5)

O PEYER'S PATCHES CONDITIONS

IRIS SIGNS:
WHITENESS IN PEYER'S PATCHES AREA
INDICATE:
FEVER DUE TO INFECTION OR INFLAMMATION
OF TONSILS, APPENDIX, CYSTITIS OR ANY OTHER
ORGAN.
DARKNESS IN PEYER'S PATCHES AREA
INDICATE:
SUPPRESSED HISTORY OF FEVERS BY DRUGS THERAPY.
(SEE ALSO FEVER PAGES F2 / F3).

O PHARYNX (SEE CHART PAGE P5)

O PILES (SEE HAEMERRHOIDS PAGE   )

O PINEAL GLAND (SEE CHART PAGE   )

O PINEAL GLAND CONDITIONS
(SEE ENDOCRINE SYSTEM CONDITIONS   )

O PITUITARY GLAND (SEE CHART PAGE   )

O PITUITARY GLAND CONDITIONS
(SEE ENDOCRINE SYSTEM CONDITIONS   )

O PLEURA AREA (SEE CHART PAGE   )

O POCKETS BOWELS (SEE BOWELS CONDITIONS   )

O POSTURE (SEE SKELETAL SYSTEM)

O PROLAPSUS (SEE BOWELS CONDITIONS)

O PROSTATE AREA (SEE CHART PAGE P5)

O PROSTATE CONDITIONS MALE

IRIS SIGNS:
DARK BOWELS AREA
BALLOONED BOWEL
DESCENDING & SIGMOID POCKETS
DARK PROSTATE AREA.

INDICATION:
CONSTIPATION
COLITIS / DIVERTICULI
CHRONIC PROSTATE CONDITION

CAUSES:
PROLONGED PRESSURE BY SIGMOID COLON ON THE
PROSTATE GLAND DUE TO CHRONIC CONSTIPATION.
ZINC DEFICIENCY.
PROLONGED SEXUAL FOREPLAY.

NOTE: WHITENESS OF PROSTATE AREA INDICATE ACUTE
INFLAMMATION AND PAIN DUE TO THE SAME CAUSES
MENTIONED ABOVE.

PROSTATE CONDITIONS

WHOLISTIC RELATIONSHIPS:
DIGESTIVE & GLANDULAR SYSTEM
DIGESTIVE & URINARY SYSTEMS
REPRODUCTIVE & URINARY SYSTEMS

TREATMENT:
TREAT CONSTIPATION
PLAIN WATER FAST
COLD WATER ENEMAS
PROSTATE FORMULA (Dr C)

AVOID: MEATS/DAIRY.
REFINED CARBOHYDRATES.

O PSORIARIS

IRIS SIGNS:
DARK BOWELS
LYMPHIC ROSARY
LYMPHIC TOPHI IN SKIN ZONE

INDICATIONS:
CONSTIPATION
LYMPHIC CONGESTION
TOXIC CIRCULATION
LYMPHIC SPILLOVER INTO SKIN ZONE

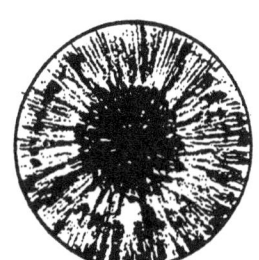

CAUSES:
CONSTIPATION AND ALL ITS CAUSES
UNDER ACTIVE SKIN, POOR PERSPIRATION
POOR ELIMINATION
TOXICITY
TOXIC BLOOD CIRCULATION
KIDNEY AND OR LIVER UNDERFUNCTION.
DAMAGE OF THE INTESTINAL WALLS

WHOLISTIC RELATIONSHIPS:
DIGESTIVE & CIRCULATORY SYSTEMS
DIGESTIVE & RESPIRATORY SYSTEMS
DIGESTIVE & LYMPHATIC SYSTEMS

TREATMENT:
ULTIMATE CLEANSING PROGRAM.   (Dr BJ).
TREAT LYMPHATIC SYSTEM.
TREAT SKIN, STIMULATE PERSPIRATION.
LIVER FLUSH, GALL BLADDER CLEANSING.
KIDNEYS CLEANSING.
EXERCISE
SKIN BRUSHING
CASTOR OIL PACKS.

O PSORIC SPOTS (SEE DRUGS SPOTS PAGE D9)
O PUPIL ABNORMALITIES
   IRIS SIGNS:
1- GREY PUPIL
   INDICATE: CATARACT
2- GREEN PUPIL
   INDICATE: GLAUCOMA.
3- PUPIL DILATION: DIRECTED BY SNS
   INDICATE:
   RESPONSE TO DARKNESS
   BEFORE EPILEPTIC FITS
   FRIGHT, EMOTIONS
   LOW MENTAL DEVELOPMENT
   BRAIN ANEMIA

4- PUPIL CONTRACTION: DIRECTED BY PNS
   INDICATE:
   RESPONSE TO BRIGHT LIGHTS
   FOCUS ON CLOSE OBJECTS
   FEVERS
   CONGESTION OF IRIS
   TENSION
5- OVAL PUPIL CONDITIONS:
   READ: FUNDAMENTAL BASIS OF IRIS DIAGNOSIS
         THEODOR KRIEGE PAGE 83
         CHAPTER 21

P CHART

P CHART TO IRIDOLOGY

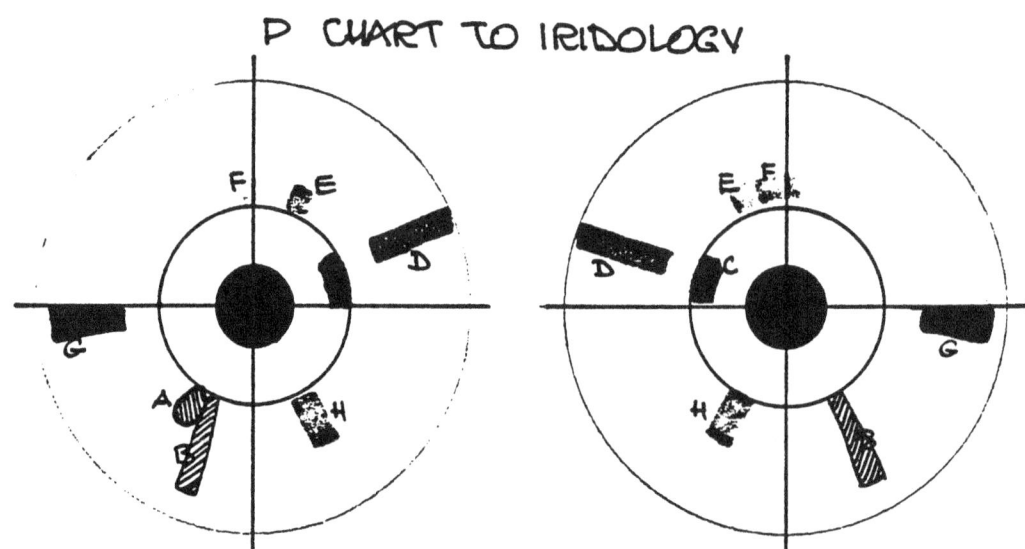

A- PANCREAS
B- PELVIS
C- PEYER'S PATCHES
D- PHARYNX

E- PINEAL GLAND
F- PITUITARY GLAND
G- PLEURA
H- PROSTATE GLAND

O RADII SOLARIS

IRIS SIGNS:
BROWN OR DARK BROWN
LINES RADIATE FROM ANW OR
PUPIL
RADII SOLARIS ALMOST OCCUR
WITH NERVE RINGS.

INDICATIONS:
CHANNELS OF TOXIC SEEPAGE
FROM THE INTESTINAL TRACT INTO
VARIOUS ORGANS OF THE BODY
AND MAINLY THE BRAIN.
THE DARKER THE COLOR, THE MORE
SERIOUS THE CONDITION.
CAUSES:
CHRONIC CONSTIPATION
PROLONGED PARASITIS INVASION
PROLONGED DIGESTIVE DISORDERS
DRUGS INTAKE EXCESS
INHERITED
IRRITATION OF CENTRAL NERVOUS SYSTEM
AND THE AUTONOMIC NERVOUS SYSTEM.
BROWN IRIS PEOPLE ARE MORE PRONE TO RADII
SOLARIS THAN BLUE IRIS PEOPLE

NOTE: RADII SOLARIS INDICATE KIDNEY FATIGUE, EVEN
THE LINES ARE NOT PASSING IN THE KIDNEY AREA
OF THE IRIS.

WHOLISTIC RELATION SHIPS.
DIGESTIVE / CIRCULATORY & ALL SYSTEMS

TREATMENTS:
ULTIMATE TISSUE CLEANSING (Dr. BJ)
STRICT VEGAN DIET
VEGETABLE BROTH FASTING
WATER FASTING
REST
TREAT NERVOUS SYSTEM
TREAT CIRCULATORY SYSTEM
AVOID VIGORIOUS EXERCISE

O RECTUM AREA (SEE CHART PAGE   )

O REPRODUCTIVE SYSTEM CONDITIONS
(SEE IMPOTANCE MALE)
(SEE INFERTILITY FEMALE.)

O REPRODUCTIVE SYSTEM AREAS
(SEE CHART PAGE R2)

REPRODUCTIVE SYSTEM

CHART TO IRIDOLOGY

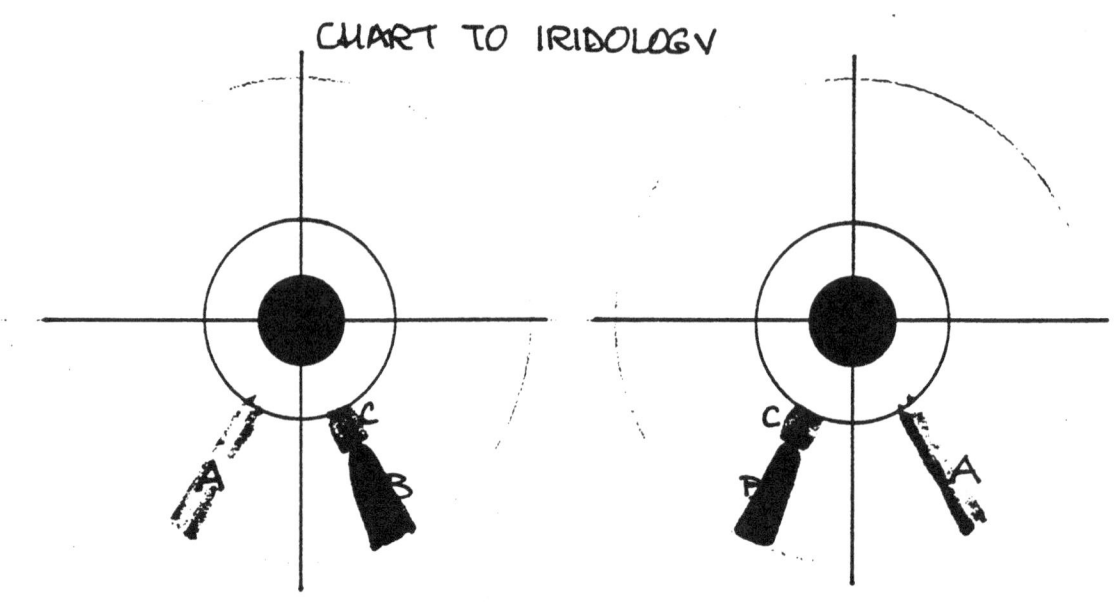

A — OVARY FEMALE
    TESTIS MALE
B — VAGINA FEMALE
    PENIS MALE
C — UTERUS FEMALE
    PROSTATE MALE

O RESPIRATORY SYSTEM CHART

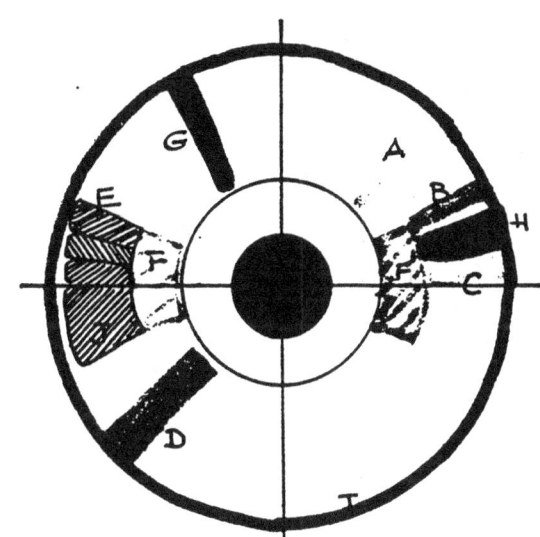 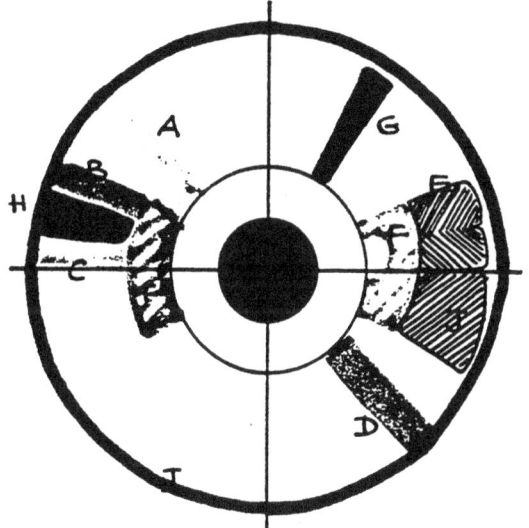

A - NOSE
B - LARYNX, PHARYNX
C - TRACHEA
D - DIAPHRAGM
E - LUNGS
F - BRONCHIALS
FI - BRONCHUS

G - MEDULLA
H - THYROID
I - LYMPH & SKIN
J - THORAX, LUNGS POSTURE

O RESPIRATORY SYSTEM CONDITIONS

(SEE BRONCHITIS PAGE B11)
(SEE LUNG CANCER PAGE C2, IRIS B)

O RHEUMATISM

IRIS SIGNS:
THICK WHITE ANW
BLUE IRIS

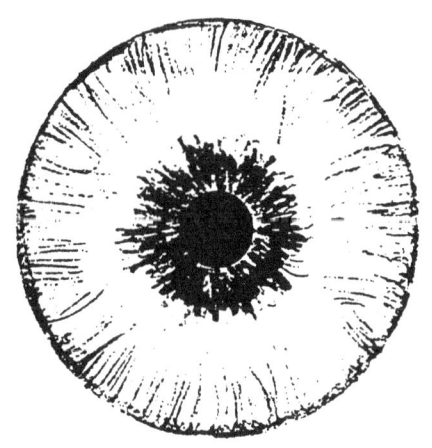

INDICATIONS:
CATARRHAL ACCUMULATION
HYPER ACIDITY
EXCESS MUCUS FORMATION
PAIN, TENSION, MUSCULAR SPASM
ARTHRITIS, BURSITIS, RHEUMATISM.

CAUSES:
SEE ACIDITY & ARTHRITIS
WHOLISTIC RELATION SHIPS:
SEE ACIDITY & ARTHRITIS

TREATMENT:
BOWELS CLEANSING
TREAT NERVOUS SYSTEM
CIRCULATION FORMULA (FD)
ALKALINE FORMULA (FD)
VEGETABLE BROTH FAST
STRICT VEGAN DIET.

O SCAPULA (SEE CHART PAGE S2)

O SCURF RIM

IRIS SIGNS:
DARKNESS AT THE PERIPHERY
OF THE IRIS
INDICATIONS:
UNDERACTIVE SKIN FUNCTION.
SLOW ELIMINATION VIA SKIN.
ACCUMULATION OF TOXIC
ELEMENTS & METABOLIC
WASTE INTO SKIN.
POOR CAPILLARY CIRCULATION.
POOR METABOLISM.
OVER LOAD TO KIDNEY.
BODY ODOR

CAUSES:
WEARING HEAVY TIGHT-FITTING
SYNTHETIC CLOTHES.
POOR SKIN VENTILATION
SUN EXPOSURE DEFICIENCY
MEATS, FATS, DAIRY EXCESS
REFINED CARBOHYDRATE EXCESS
LACK OF PHYSICAL EXERCISE
DEODORENT & LOTIONS USE.
CONSTIPATION.

WHOLISTIC RELATION SHIPS:
CIRCULATORY & LYMPHATIC SYSTEMS
CIRCULATORY & RESPIRATORY SYSTEMS
CIRCULATORY & URINARY SYSTEMS

TREATMENT:
BOWELS CLEANSING.
STIMULATE SKIN FUNCTION.
SUN BATHING, AIR BATHING, SAUNA, SWIMMING.
SKIN BRUSHING.
EXERCISE.
FENUGREEK.
TREAT ALSO LYMPHIC SYSTEM.

O SENSES FIVE SENSE AREA (SEE CHART PAGE S6)

O SENILITY (SEE ARCUS SENILIS)

O SEX LIFE CENTER (SEE CHART PAGE S6)

O SEX ORGANS (SEE CHART PAGE S6)

O SHOULDER (SEE CHART PAGE S6)

O SIGMOID COLON (SEE CHART PAGE S6)

O SIGMOID COLON CONDITIONS
(SEE CONSTIPATION)
(SEE BOWELS CONDITIONS)

O SINUS CONDITIONS

IRIS SIGNS:
YELLOW-ORANGE DISCOLORATIONS
IN THE UPPER IRIS AREA RADIATING
FROM ANW.
DARK BOWELS AREA.

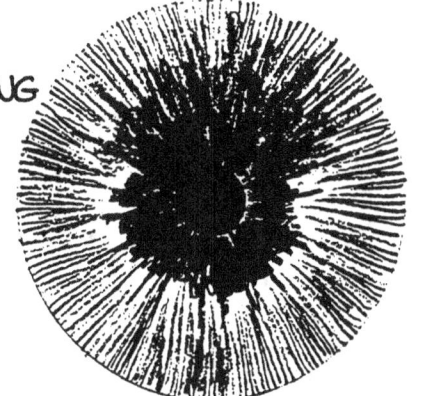

INDICATIONS:
TOXINS RADIATING FROM THE
TRANSVERSE COLON INTO HEAD
AREA.
CONSTIPATION
SINUSITIS.

CAUSES:
CONSTIPATION & FAECES ACCUMULATION IN THE TRANSVERSE
COLON.
PINEAL & PITUITARY AFFECTED.
EARS, EYES & NOSE AFFECTED.

WHOLISTIC RELATION SHIPS:
CIRCULATORY & DIGESTIVE SYSTEMS
CIRCULATORY & ENDOCRINE SYSTEMS
CIRCULATORY & RESPIRATORY SYSTEMS.

TREATMENT:
TREAT CONSTIPATION.
TREAT ACIDITY.
TREAT LYMPHATIC SYSTEM.

O SKELETAL SYSTEM CHART

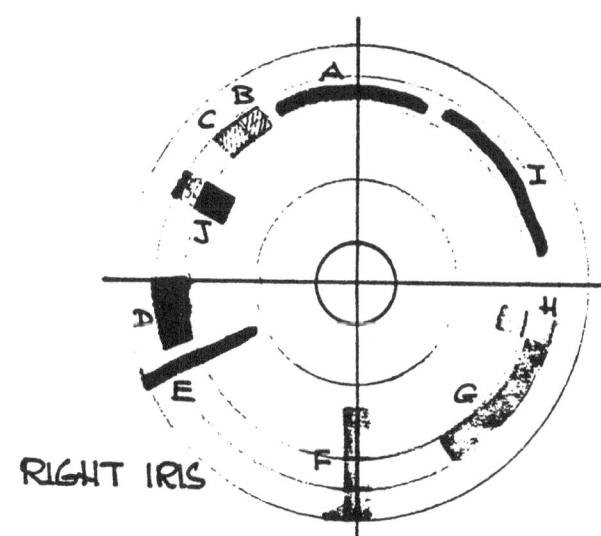

RIGHT IRIS

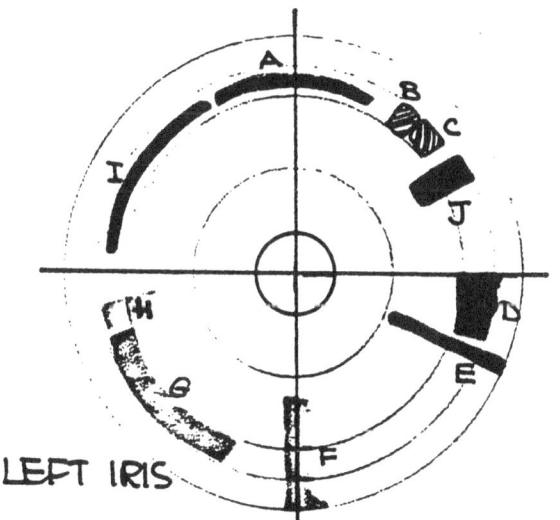

LEFT IRIS

A_CRANIAL BONES
B_EAR
C_CERVICAL VERTEBRAE
D_CHEST RIBS
E_HAND
F_FOOT & LEG

G_BACK : SPINAL BONES
H_SCAPULA
I_FACIAL BONES AND
   TEETH
J_SHOULDER & CLEVICLE.

O SKELETAL SYSTEM CONDITIONS

1_ DARKNESS IN SKELETAL AREAS
INDICATE: POOR POSTURE
CALCIUM DEFICIENCY
2_ DARK SPOTS IN BONE, SKIN AND LYMPH AREAS.
INDICATE: OSTEOPOROSIS
3_ RAISED WHITE FIBRES IN SPINE AREA.
INDICATE: BONE INFLAMMATION & PAIN.
4_ LYMPHATIC TOPHI IN THE SKELETAL AREA.
INDICATE: INFLAMMATION AROUND BONE AREA.
5_ DISCOLORATION IN THE PARATHYROID GLAND AREA.
INDICATE: HYPO OR HYPERFUNTION OF THE PARA-
THYROID GLAND CAUSING CALCIUM SODIUM IMBALANCE.
6_ SODIUM RING IN THE SKELETAL AREA.
INDICATE: CALCIUM DEPOSITS IN BLOOD STREEM
AND CALCIUM MALABSORBTION.
7_ DARKNESS & NERVE RINGS IN THE LOWER BACK
AREA.
INDICATE: SPINAL LESIONS AFFECTING KIDNEYS
AND BLADDER.
8_ THICK WHITE ANW.
INDICATE: TENDENCY TO ARTHRITIS, BURSITIS, GOUT
AND RHEOMATISM.

O SKIN AREA (SEE RESPIRATORY SYSTEM'S CHART)
O SKIN CONDITIONS
SEE SCURF RIM
SEE ANEMIA
SEE PSORIARIS
SEE ACNE
SEE BOILS
SEE CANCER
SEE CIRCULATORY SYSTEM
SEE PERSPIRATION

O SMALL INTESTINES AREA
(SEE DIGESTIVE SYSTEM CHART)

O SODIUM RING
IRIS SIGNS:
WHITENERS & LOSS OF FIBERS
IN THE CILIARY ZONE
INDICATIONS:
CALCIUM DEPOSITS
SODIUM EXCESS
CHOLESTEROLE DEPOSITING
HARDNING OF ARTERIES
AGEING, ARTERIOSCLEROSIS

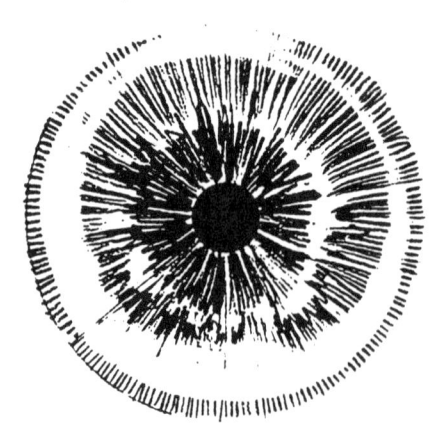

SODIUM RING

CAUSES:
RICH SALTED CHEESE EXCESS
PICKELS EXCESS
PROCESSED & CANNED MEATS
SODIUM EXCESS
CONSTIPATION, POOR ELIMINATION
FATS EXCESS
MINERALS IMBALANCES
HYPER ACIDITY IN YOUNG AGES.
WHOLISTIC RELATION SHIPS:
CIRCULATORY & DIGESTIVE SYSTEMS
CIRCULATORY & SKELETAL SYSTEMS.
CIRCULATORY & MUSCULAR SYSTEMS

TREATMENT:
ACID ALKALINE BALANCING
VEGETABLE JUICES
TREAT CHOLESTEROLE
TREAT CONSTIPATION
TREAT CIRCULATORY SYSTEM

O SOLAR PLEXUS (SEE CHART PAGE S6)

O SPASM (SEE ACIDITY PAGE A1)

O SPASTIC COLON (SEE BOWELS CONDITIONS, STRICTURE)

O SPEACH CENTER AREA (SEE CHART PAGE S6)

O SPINAL BONES (SEE CHART PAGE S2)

O SPLEEN AREA (SEE CHART PAGE S6)

O SPLEEN CONDITIONS

A_ SPENITIS
IRIS SIGNS:
LIGHTENING OF THE SPLEEN AREA.
INDICATE: INFLAMMATION OF THE SPLEEN.

B_ LYMPHIC CONGESTION
IRIS SIGNS:
WHITE_YELLOW_BROWN TOPHI IN THE CIRCULATORY ZONE.
INDICATE: UNDER FUNCTION OF THE LYMPH & SPLEEN.

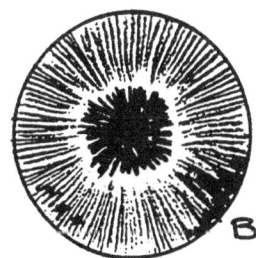

LEFT IRIS

C_ SPLEEN HYPOFUNCTION
IRIS SIGNS:
BLACK OR DARK BROWN LINES OR RADII SOLARIS IN SPLEEN AREA.
INDICATE: TOXIC SEEPAGE FROM BOWELS VIA BLOOD STREAM INTO SPLEEN.

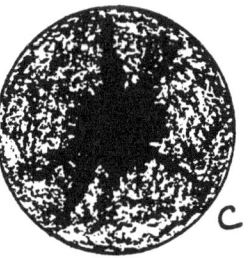

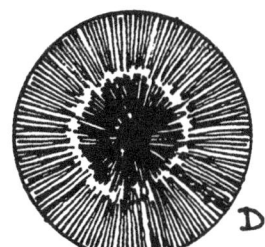

D_ SPLEEN TUMOUR.
DARK POINTS IN SPLEEN AREA.
INDICATE: A MALIGNANT CONDITION OF SPLEEN AND POSSIBILITY TO TUMOUR.

SPLEEN CONDITIONS

CAUSES:
CONSTIPATION
UNTREATED LYMPHATIC CONGESTION IN ITS ACUTE AND
    SUB ACUTE STAGES.
LIVER CONGESTION.
TOXIC BLOOD.
PROLONGED ANTIBIOTICS & VARIOUS DRUGS.
FRESH FRUITS & VEGETABLES DEFICIENCY.
POOR BLOOD CIRCULATION
LACK OF PHYSICAL EXERCISE.

WHOLISTIC RELATIONSHIPS.
LYMPHIC & CIRCULATORY SYSTEMS
LYMPHIC & DIGESTIVE SYSTEMS
LYMPHIC & NERVOUS SYSTEMS.

TREATMENT:
TREAT CONSTIPATION.
TREAT CIRCULATION.
TREAT LYMPHIC SYSTEM
TREAT NERVOUS SYSTEM.

O STOMACH AREA (SEE DIGESTIVE SYSTEM CHART)
O STOMACH CONDITIONS
IRIS SIGNS:
1. WHITE STOMACH RING
INDICATE:
HYPER ACID STOMACH (SEE ACID STOMACH PAGE   )
2. DARK BROWN STOMACH RING
INDICATE:
UNDERACID STOMACH
HCL DEFICIENCY.
3. GASTRITIS. (SEE GASTRITIS PAGE   )

O STOMACH ULCER
IRIS SIGNS:
BLACK SPOT IN STOMACH AREA CLOSE TO
PUPIL & ANW.
RAISED WHITE FIBERS AROUND THE
SPOT & RADIATING TOWARDS THE
CILIARY ZONE.
INDICATIONS:
DAMAGE BY ULCEROUS CONDITION
OF THE STOMACH WALL.
PAIN IN STOMACH AND BODY
ORGANS CLOSE IN RELATION WITH
ANW.

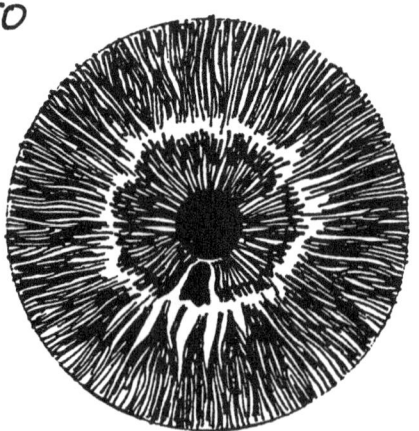

CAUSES:
PROLONGED UNTREATED CONDITION
OF HYPO/OR HYPERACID STOMACH.
CONSTIPATION WITH ALL ITS CAUSES.
PROLONGED TENSION AND PERMAMENT EMOTIONAL
STRESS.
NERVOUS IRRITATION.
FRUSTRATIONS.

STOMACH ULCER

WHOLISTIC RELATION SHIPS:
DIGESTIVE & NERVOUS SYSTEMS
DIGESTIVE & CIRCULATORY SYSTEMS
DIGESTIVE & MUSCULAR SYSTEMS.

TREATMENT:
TREAT CONSTIPATION.
ACID/ALKALINE BALANCING FORMULA (FD).
RAW CARROT JUICE.
RAW CABBAGE JUICE.
RAW POTATO JUICE.
TREAT NERVOUS SYSTEM.
MACROBIOTIC DIET.

S CHART TO IRIDOLOGY

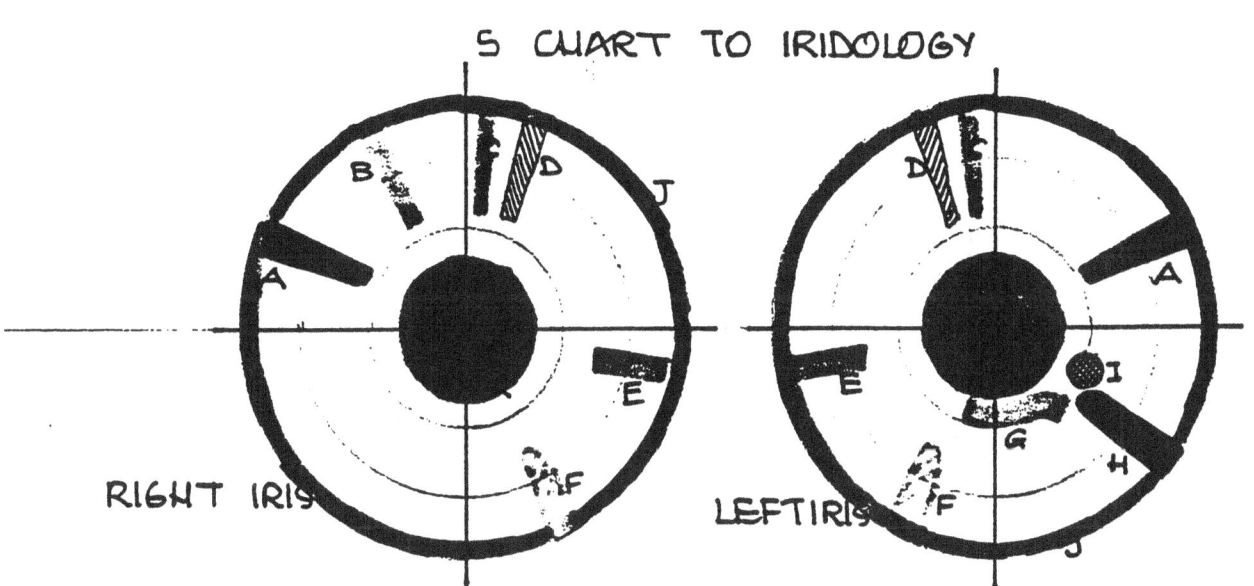

RIGHT IRIS   LEFT IRIS

A — SHOULDER
B — SEX IMPULSE AREA
C — SENSE AREA (5 SENSES)
D — SPEECH AREA
E — SCAPULA
F — SEX ORGAN (VAGINA/PENIS)
G — SIGMOID COLON
H — SPLEEN
I — SOLAR PEXUS
J — SKIN
K — STOMACH

O TENSION

IRIS SIGNS:
SMALL PUPIL.
CONTRACTED ANW.
DARK THYROID.
NERVE RINGS IN
 LYMPHIC ZONE.
WHITE EGO PRESSURE
 AREA.

(NOTE: THESE SIGNS MAY NOT
 EXIST ALL TOGETHER IN ONE
 IRIS AT THE SAME TIME.)

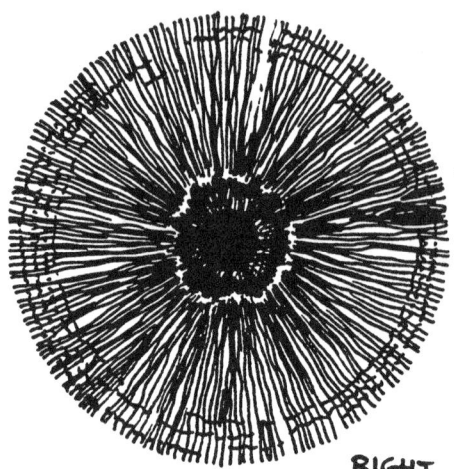

RIGHT

INDICATIONS:
PNS / SNS IMBALANCE.
IODINE DEFICIENCY.
NERVOUS IRRITATION.
TENDENCY TO HIGH BLOOD PRESSURE
VERY HIGH TENDENCY TO TENSION.

CAUSES:
IRRITATED AUTONOMIC NERVOUS SYSTEM.
IRRITATED CENTRAL NERVOUS SYSTEM.
HYPER ACIDITY.
POTASSIUM / MAGNESIUM DEFICIENCY.
PLASTIC LIFE STYLE.
LIVING IN HIGH BUILDINGS (TOWERS)
COFFEE / TEA, TOBACO, ALCOHOLS.
HYPOGLYCEMIA.
PERFECTIONISTS.
BAD BREATHING QUALITY.

WHOLISTIC RELATION SHIPS.
NERVOUS & CIRCULATORY SYSTEMS.
NERVOUS & DIGESTIVE SYSTEMS.
NERVOUS & MUSCULAR SYSTEMS.
NERVOUS & ENDOCRINE SYSTEMS.

TREATMENT:
TREAT NERVOUS SYSTEM
ACID / ALKALINE BALANCING
BOWELS CLEANSING.
TREAT THYROID / ADRENAL GLANDS.
BREATHING EXERCISE.
YOGA / MEDITATION.
WALKING BAREFEET.
SWIMMING, JOGGING.
VEGETABLE BROTH.
RAW FRESH VEGETABLES.

O TESTES AREA (SEE CHART PAGE T6)
O THIGH AREA (SEE CHART PAGE T6)
O THROAT AREA (SEE CHART PAGE T6)
O THYMUS GLAND AREA (SEE CHART PAGE T6)
O THYMUS GLAND CONDITIONS (CHILDREN)

IRIS SIGNS:
WHITE_YELLOW_ORANGE THYMUS AREA
INDICATE:
TOXIC CONDITION OF THYMUS GLAND.
DIMINISHED GLANDULAR FUNCTION.
FREQUENT COLDS & INFECTIONS.
POOR IMMUNITY.
SLOW RECOVERY.

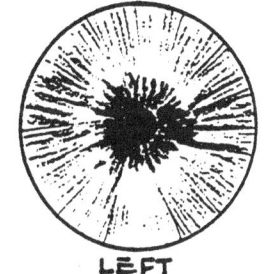
LEFT

CAUSES:
INHERITED WEAKNESS.
REFINED CARBOHYDRATES EXCESS
 CHOCOLETS/CONFECTIONARIES/DONUTS ECT.
CANNED POWDERED MILK.
EARLY WEANING
MOTHER'S MILK DEFICIENCY.

WHOLISTIC RELATION SHIPS:
ENDOCRINE & LYMPHATIC SYSTEMS.
ENDOCRINE & CIRCULATORY SYSTEMS.
ENDOCRINE & DIGESTIVE SYSTEMS.

TREATMENT:
ALMONDS MILK IS AN EXCELLENT BALANCED MINERAL
 AND ALKALINIC PROTEIN.
VEGETABLE BROTH FAST.
FRESH RAW FRUITS.

O THYROID GLAND AREA (SEE CHART PAGE T6)
O THYROID GLAND CODITIONS
IRIS SIGNS:
A_ WHITE THYROID AREA
   THICK WHITE ANW.
INDICATION:
   HYPER THYROIDISM.
   HIGH METABOLIC RATE.
   OVER ACTIVITY. ACUTE STAGE

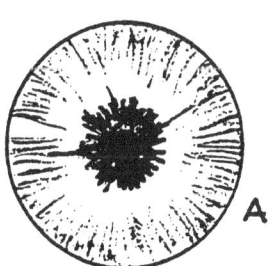
A

B_ YELLOW BROWN THYROID AREA
  ORANG_BROWN ANW.
INDICATION:
   TOXIC THYROID, SUB ACUTE STAGE
   TOXIC BLOOD SUPPLY, CONSTIPATION.
   THYROID DIMINISHED FUNCTION.

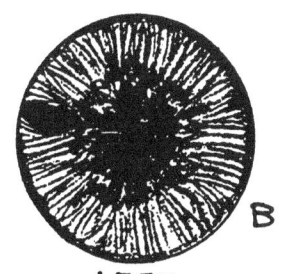
B
LEFT

THYROID CONDITIONS

C – DARK THYROID AREA
    DARK ADRENAL
    DARK BOWELS/DARK STOMACH RING.
    ARCUS SENILIS
    COARSE FIBERS.

INDICATIONS:
    HYPOTHYROIDISM.
    UNDER FUNCTION ADRENAL.
    CONSTIPATION.
    UNDER ACID STOMACH.
    BRAIN ANEMIA.
    POOR CONSTITUTION.
    IODINE/CALCIUM DEFICIENCY.
    GOITER.
    POOR METABOLIC FUNCTION.
    PINEAL & PITUITARY AFFECTED.

CAUSES:
    UNTREATED ACUTE STAGES OF DISEASE
    SUPPRESSED TONSILITIS.
    CONSTIPATION.
    IODINE DEFICIENCY
    PITUITARY DISORDERS
    SUPPRESSED LYMPHIC DISORDERS
    VITAMINES/MINERALS DEFICIENCY.
    ENDOCRINE IMBALANCES.

WHOLISTIC RELATIONSHIPS:
    ENDOCRINE & DIGESTIVE SYSTEMS.
    ENDOCRINE & CIRCULATORY SYSTEMS.
    ENDOCRINE & LYMPHIC SYSTEMS.

LEFT   C

TREATMENT:
    BLOOD PURIFYING   (PD).
    BLOOD CIRCULATION (FD).
    THYROID FORMULA (FD).
    KELP.
    MULTI MINERAL/VITAMINS NATURAL (PD).
    TREAT CONSTIPATION.
    TREAT SINUSITIS.
    TREAT LYMPH.
    TREAT HYPOGLYCEMIA.
    TREAT ELIMINATIVE CHANNELS.
    RAW FRESH FRUITS & VEGETABLES.
    EXERCISE.

O TONGUE AREA (SEE CHART PAGE T6)
O TONSILS AREA (SEE CHART PAGE T6)

○ TONSILS CONDITIONS

1_ IRIS SIGNS:
  WHITE TONSILS
  WHITE PEYER'S PATCHES.

  INDICATE:
  ACUTE TONSILITIS
  FEVER
  PAIN.

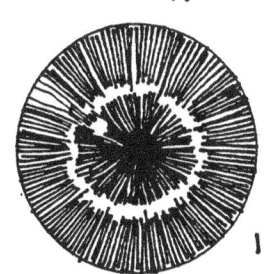

LEFT.

1

2_ IRIS SIGNS:
  LYMPHIC ROSARY (YELLOW_ORANGE)
  WHITE PEYER'S PATCHES.
  ORANG_BROWN CLOUDS IN TONSILS AREA.

  INDICATE:
  SUB_ACUTE TONSILITIS.
  LYMPHIC CONGESTION.
  FEVERS, PAIN,
  SLOW RECOVERY.
  POOR IMMUNITY.

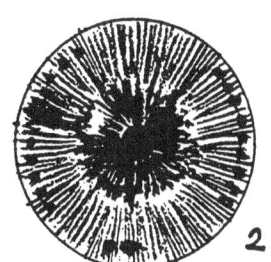

2

3_ IRIS SIGNS:
  DARK TONSILS AREA
  DARK ANW / BOWEL AREA.
  DARK BROWN LYMPHIC ROSARY
  NERVE RINGS.
  DARK SPLEEN
  WEAKNESS LESIONS IN LUNGS AREA.

  INDICATE:
  CHRONIC_DEGENERATIVE STAGE
   OF TONSILS.
  CONSTIPATION.
  CHRONIC LYMPH CONGESTION.
  METABOLIC IRRITATION.
  SPLEEN CONGESTION.
  POOR BREATHING.

3

CAUSES:
  HYPERACIDITY.
  LYMPHIC CONGESTION
  POTASSIUM, MAGNESIUM, SODIUM, CALCIUM DEFICIENCY.
  MEATS, FATS, DAIRY, SUGARS, FRIED FOODS, BREAD.
  POOR ELIMINATIONS.
  POOR SKIN FUNCTION.
  CONSTIPATION.
  STRESS AND DEPRESSIONS (DUE TO B FAMILY AND C_
   VITAMINS INCREDIBLE LOSSES) CAUSED BY SCHOOLS
   AND TEACHERS, AND STUPID CRUEL EXAMINATIONS.

TONSILS CONDITIONS.

WHOLISTIC RELATION SHIPS:

LYMPHIC & CIRCULATORY SYSTEMS
LYMPHIC & DIGESTIVE SYSTEMS
LYMPHIC & RESPIRATORY SYSTEMS
LYMPHIC & NERVOUS SYSTEMS.

TREATMENTS:
BOWELS CLEANSING
BLOOD PURIFICATION (FD)
STIMULATE ELIMINATIONS
AIR BATHINGS, SKIN BRUSHING.
TREAT LYMPHIC SYSTEM.
VEGETABLES BROTH FAST.
ALKALINE FORMULA (FD)
ACID/ALKALINE BALANCING
REST.

PREVENTIVE MEASURES:
 STRICT VEGAN DIET.
 DAILY FRESH RAW F VEGETABLES. (LEAVES)
 WHOLE RICE, WHOLE WHEAT.
 ALMONDS, DRIED FRUITS.
 WARM WATER WITH LEMON BEFORE BREAKFAST.

AVOID:
 MILK.
 DAIRY, MEATS, FATS, FRIED FOODS.
 ROASTED PEANUT
 PEANUT BUTTER.
 SWEETS, BREAD, BEVERAGES.
 CANNED FOOD
 FOOD ADDITIVES, COLORINGS, FLAVORINGS.

O TOXIC ABSORBTION (SEE CIRCULATORY DISEASES)
O TOXIC SETTLEMENTS (SEE DRUG SPOTS)
O TRANSVERSE COLON (SEE CHART PAGE T6)
O TRANSVERSE COLON CONDITIONS
 (SEE PROLAPSUS PAGE   )
 (SEE ENDOCRINE DISORDERS PAGE   )
 (SEE SINUS CONDITIONS PAGE   )

CHART TO IRIDOLOGY

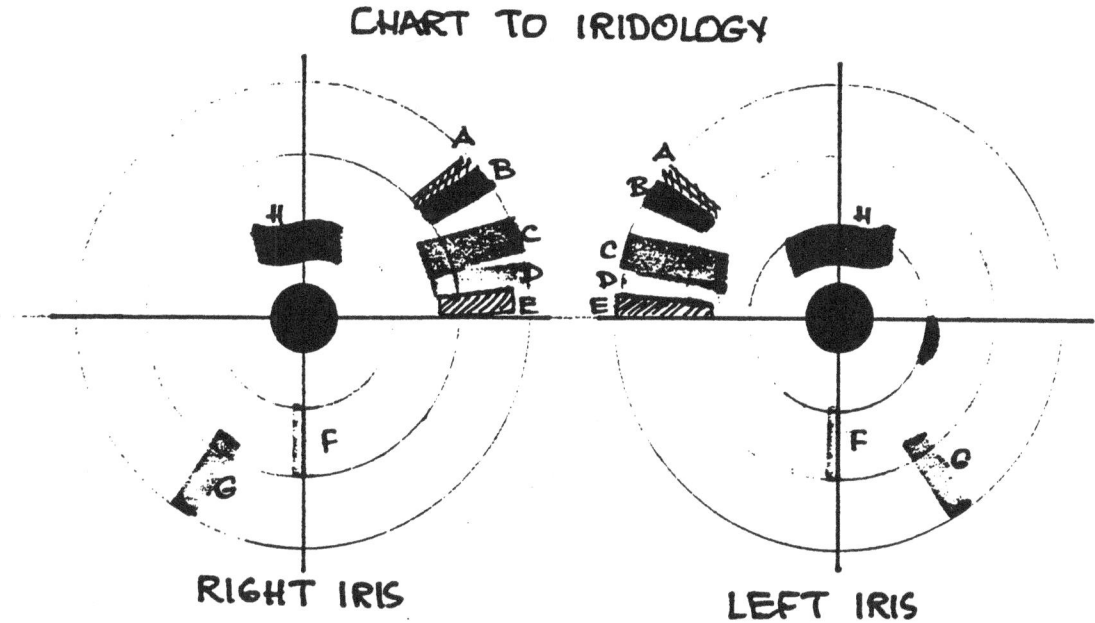

RIGHT IRIS   LEFT IRIS

A - TONGUE
B - TONSILS
C - THYROID GLAND
D - THROAT
E - TRACHEA
F - THIGH
G - TESTES.
H - TRANSVERSE COLON (SEE ALSO DIGESTIVE SYSTEM)

O ULCERS
  DUODENAL ULCER (PAGE   )
  GASTRIC ULCER (SEE STOMACH ULCERS PAGE   )
O URETHRA (SEE URNARY CHART)
O URIC ACID (SEE GOUT PAGE   )
O URINARY SYSTEM CHART

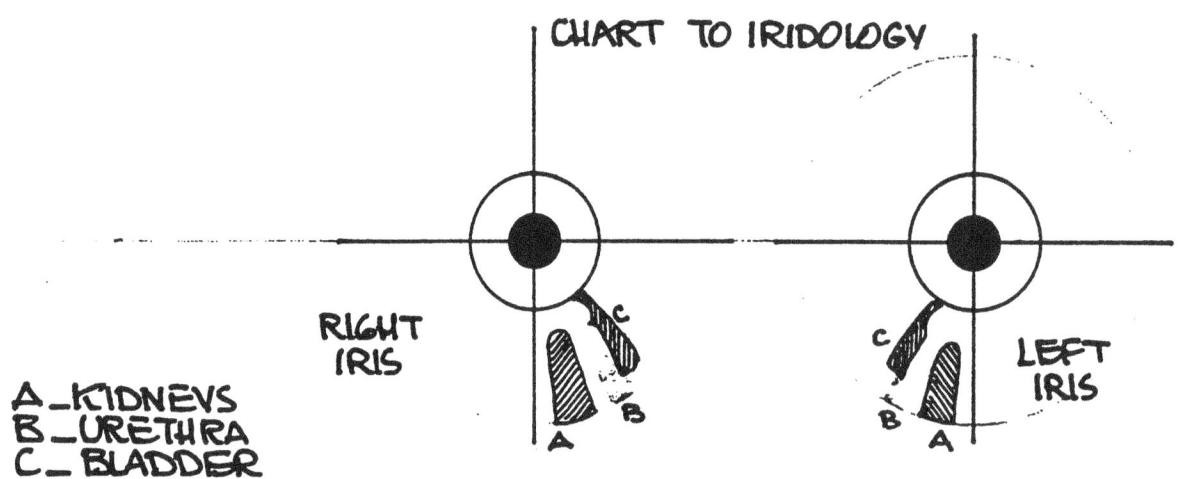

CHART TO IRIDOLOGY

RIGHT IRIS

LEFT IRIS

A – KIDNEYS
B – URETHRA
C – BLADDER

O URINARY SYSTEM CONDITIONS
  (SEE BLADDER CONDITIONS PAGE B4)
  (SEE KIDNEY CONDITIONS PAGE K1)

O UTERUS AREA
  (SEE REPRODUCTIVE SYSTEM CHART PAGE   )

O VAGINAL AREA (SEE CHART PAGE   )
O VAGINAL CONDITIONS

A_ IRIS SIGNS:
WHITE VAGINAL / UTERUS AREAS.
SCURF RIM.
ORANGE BROWN ANW.

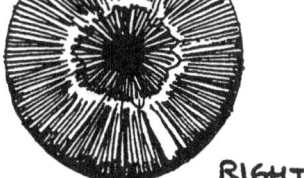

RIGHT.

INDICATIONS:
ACUTE VAGINITIS.
PUS.
POOR VENTILATION AND SKIN
  UNDERFUNCTION IN THE GENITO_URINARY ORGANS.
CONSTIPATION AND TOXIC BLOOD SUPPLY.

CAUSES:
CONSTIPATION AND ALL ITS DIETERY CAUSES.
ANTIBIOTICS.
TOXICITY.
CYSTITIS.
POOR HYGIENE.
TIGHT_FITTING SYNTHETIC UNDERWEAR.
MOIST ENVIRONMENT.
POOR PERSPIRATION.
SKIN DISORDERS.

WHOLISTIC RELATION SHIPS
REPRODUCTIVE & URINARY SYSTEMS
REPRODUCTIVE & DIGESTIVE SYSTEMS
REPRODUCTIVE / URINARY & CIRCULATORY SYSTEMS
REPRODUCTIVE / URINARY & RESPIRATORY SYSTEMS.

TREATMENT:

TREAT CONSTIPATION.
BLOOD PURIFICATION (FD).
BLOOD CIRCULATION (FD).
VAGINAL BOLUS (FD).
KIDNEY FLUSHING.
STIMULATE SKIN FUNCTION.
STIMULATE ALL ELIMINATIVE ORGANS.
C VITAMIN NATURAL SOURCES
B6 VITAMIN NATURAL SOURCES.
FRESH RAW LEAFY VEGETABLES

O VARICOSE VEINS

IRIS SIGNS:
SCURF RIM
WHITE & BLACK LINES IN LEG AREA
INDICATE:
ULCERATED CONDITION OF
  VARICOSE VEINS.
STAGNANT CAPILLARY CIRCULATION.

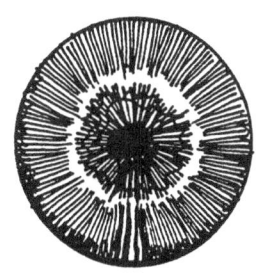

VARICOSE VEINS

CAUSES:
CONSTIPATION.
POOR CIRCULATION.
LACK OF EXERCISE.
PROLONGED STANDING.
LIVER DISORDERS.
PREGNANCY.

WHOLISTIC RELATION SHIPS:
CIRCULATORY & DIGESTIVE SYSTEMS
CIRCULATORY & NERVOUS SYSTEMS.

TREATMENT:
BOWELS CLEANSING.
LIVER FLUSHING.
BLOOD CIRCULATION.
VEGETABLES BROTH FAST.
WATER FAST.
SLANT BOARD TIP-U-UP.
MASSAGES
WALKING BARE FEET.

O VEINS AREA (SEE CHART PAGE   )
O VITAMINS DEFICIENCIES
  △ VITAMIN: IRIS SIGNS:
        WHITE STOMACH RING (ACID STOMACH)
        WHITE LUNGS (ACUTE MUCUS MEMBRANES)
        DARK EYE AREA (POOR RETINAL WALL)
        FLOWER PATTERN ANW.
        DARK LIVER / ULCERS SIGNS.
  B FAMILY VITAMINS: IRIS SIGNS:
        DARK BOWELS (CONSTIPATION)
        ARCUS SINILIS (ANEMIA CONDITIONS)
        SCURF RIM (POOR METABOLISM)
        DARK LIVER / DARK KIDNEYS / DARK SPLEEM.
        INSOMNIA SIGNS / DEPRESSION SIGNS.

  C VITAMIN, IRIS SIGNS:
        (SEE OXYGENATION PAGE 02)
        DARKNESS / COARSE FIBERS (SCURVY)
        DARK MOUTH (PYORRHEA)
        ULCERS SIGNS / ANEMIA SIGNS / SCURF RIM.
        SODIUM RING (CHOLESTEROLE / ARTERIOSCLEROSIS)

  D VITAMIN: IRIS SIGNS:
        DARK BONES AREA (POOR CALCIUM)
        SODIUM RING (CALCIUM DEPOSITS)
        SCURF RIM (SUN EXPOSURE DEFICIENCY)
        HEART / AORTA CONDITIONS.
  E VITAMIN: IRIS SIGNS:
        (SEE OXYGEN DEFICIENCY PAGE 02)
        SODIUM RING / SCURF RIM / VARICOSIS SIGNS.
        ARCUS SENILIS / ATROPHY SIGNS
        DARK TESTES / DARK ANW.

O WEAKNESS SIGNS

1. WEAKNESS LESIONS:
   A — ASPARAGUS
   B — BUTTERFLY
   C — CLOSED LESION
   D — OPENED LESION
   E — DIAMOND
   F — LEAF LESION
   G — MEDUSSA
   H — LANCE

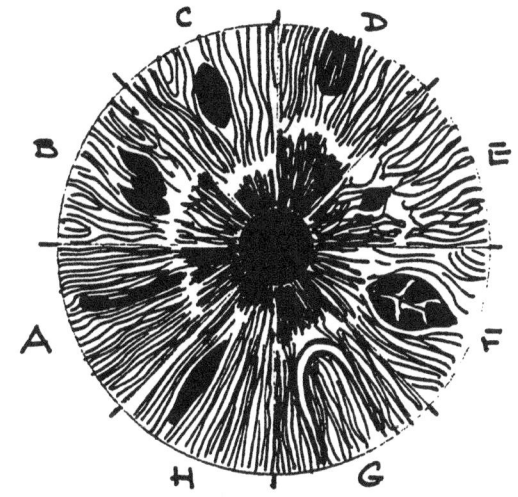

2. WEAKNESS CONDITIONS:
   ANEMIA RINGS / ARCUS SENILIS
   ANEMIA AT THE EXTREMITIES
   SODIUM RING
   NERVE RINGS
   SCURF RIM
   RADII SOLARIS
   PSORIC SPOTS
   ANW ABNORMALITIES / PUPIL ABNORMALITIES.
   DARKNESS / HETEROCHROMIA.
   FLOWER PATTERNS

O WILL POWER AREA
FROM ANW TO UPPER IRIS RIM AT 12

O WILL POWER CONDITIONS

1 — SILK PATTERNS:
   NATURAL, INSTINCTIVE, STRONG
   WILL POWER.
2 — WHITE FIBERS:
   GOOD WILL POWER DUE TO
   A HYPERACTIVE CONDITION.
3 — ORANG-BROWN LESIONS:
   SLUGGISHNESS
   WILL POWER PRETENDED ONLY
   NOT REAL.
4 — DARKNESS:
   PERMANENT LOSS OF VITALITY
   AND WILL POWER.

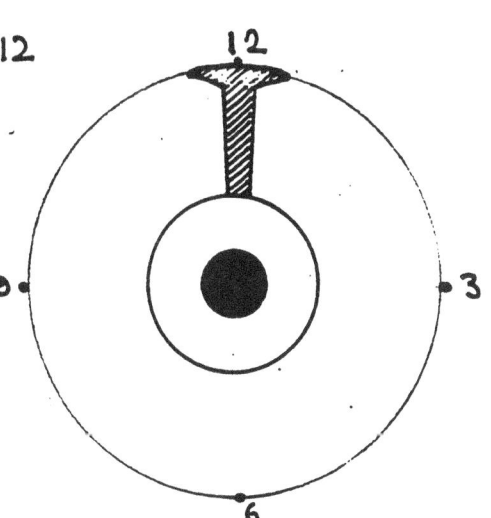

BIBLIOGRAPHY

1 — BRITISH SCHOOL OF IRIDOLOGY
   CORRESPONDENCE COURSE
          BY
   Dr. FARIDA SHARAN
2 — HERBS OF GRACE   BY Dr. FARIDA SHARAN
3 — THE SCIENCE AND PRACTICE OF IRIDOLOGY
   BY Dr. BERNARD JENSEN.
4 — IRIDOLOGY — SCIENCE AND PRCTICE
   IN THE HEALING ARTS VOL II
   BY Dr. BERNARD JENSEN.
5 — IRIDOLOGY BY DOROTHY HALL.
6 — FUNDAMENTAL BASIS OF IRISDIAGNOSIS
   BY THEODOR KRIEGE.
7 — TISSUE CLEANSING THROUGH BOWEL MANAGMENT
   BY Dr. BERNARD JENSEN.
8 — BETTER HEALTH THROUGH NATURAL HEALING
   BY ROSS TRATTLER.
9 — CANCER PREVENTION DIET
   BY: MICHIO KUSHI
10 — MANY BOOKS FROM THORSONS
11 — OWN EXPERIENCE.

www.ingramcontent.com/pod-product-compliance
Lightning Source LLC
Chambersburg PA
CBHW080950290526
45795CB00009B/2952